"This book is an offering and intervention that unearths the brutal legacy of violent ideologies and practices underpinning the field of 'mental health' while illuminating the path for mental health practitioners to reclaim our collective humanity. St. Aime takes us on a sacred journey of disruption, transformation and embodiment in this powerful work. May we commit to unlearning and divesting from oppressive systems to seed collective liberation."

Erica Woodland, *LCSW founding director of National Queer & Trans Therapists of Color Network and co-author of Healing Justice Lineages: Dreaming at the Crossroads of Liberation, Collective Care, and Safety*

"Be ready for this extraordinary book to engage you in a way that others have not. Beneath its brilliant prose and broadly incisive analysis, this book offers an invitation into something even more profound: a new way of being present. While reading it, I felt an earth-rattling resonance with its spellbinding song of vulnerability, rootedness, heartbreak, unlearning, radical embodiment, and an utterly clear-eyed sense of possibility. And I felt it throughout all of me. Something we deeply need waits within these pages."

Bill Brennan, *PhD, author of EMBARK Psychedelic Therapy: A New Approach for the Whole Person*

"Florie St. Aime is a pioneer in the mental health field. Any mental health professional who is willing to expand their awareness beyond traditional psychology will find the embodied concepts in 'Unlearning' extremely useful as they hold a healing, liberating, sympathetic space for themselves and their clients."

Kylea Taylor, *author of The Ethics of Caring, Founder of InnerEthics®*

Anti-Oppressive Psychotherapeutic Practice

This book supports mental health practitioners in showing how they personally intersect with oppression, helping them explore how it shows up in their practice and providing them with tools to offer anti-oppressive care.

Written in an accessible and spiritual tone, chapters discuss the human need for connection as well as demonstrate the oppression through a social, neuroscientific, and biological lens as something that resides and can be passed on generationally. St. Aime interrogates the idea of the moral cloak symbiotic with whiteness and encourages readers to separate themselves from their profession to become a reflective rather than defensive clinician. She defines anti-oppressive practice as a clinical approach that considers the systemic, intergenerational, sociocultural and political influences on the lives of individuals and identifies the pillars of anti-oppressive practice as interconnectedness, interdependence, boundless curiosity, and vulnerability. With chapters including both experimental and practical exercises to use with clients as well as alone, this book encourages clinicians to undergo the process of unlearning the internalized oppressions that exist within themselves to change the therapeutic power exchange and provide the best care possible.

This book is essential reading for clinical social workers in practice and in training, as well as for psychotherapists, counselors, marriage and family therapists, and other mental health practitioners.

Florie St. Aime (she/her) is a Licensed Clinical Social Worker from Brooklyn, NY, and describes herself as a liberation-based clinician. She invites others into liberation practices through organizing/activism, group facilitation/workshops, counseling, holding sacred space and clinical supervision.

Anti-Oppressive Psychotherapeutic Practice

Finding Liberation Through Unlearning

Florie St. Aime

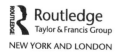

Routledge
Taylor & Francis Group

NEW YORK AND LONDON

Designed cover image: Kelli Prescott

First published 2025
by Routledge
605 Third Avenue, New York, NY 10158

and by Routledge
4 Park Square, Milton Park, Abingdon, Oxon OX14 4RN

Routledge is an imprint of the Taylor & Francis Group, an informa business

© 2025 Florie St. Aime

ISBN: 978-1-032-07461-0 (hbk)
ISBN: 978-1-032-07459-7 (pbk)
ISBN: 978-1-003-20705-4 (ebk)

DOI: 10.4324/9781003207054

Typeset in Times New Roman
by Apex CoVantage, LLC

For
RL

Contents

An Offering

Learning.

I am learning so much every moment of the day.

I am learning how I am feeling. How things impact me. Learning to feel the gait of my walk. Learning to hear the sound of my own voice. Learning strategies to survive capitalism; learning my imagination can stretch to a world post-capitalism and into thriving.

Learning I am nature. Learning my right proportion in nature.

And learning my craft. Learning what it means to sit for others. Learning theories that others have created and tested. Learning my unique skill of interpretation and practice.

And because this learning is never-ending, writing a book does not seem right. A book feels so definitive. So authoritative, so expert. And there is no way I can be an expert when I literally feel myself learning, growing and adapting every single day.

But that is not what a book is for, is it?

It is not about expertise as much as it is an offering. I have been fed by the offerings of many. Their offerings have changed meaning as I have changed, and it is with this in mind I make this offering to you.

I write because I am offering what I have up to this point in hopes that as you read, as you change, my offerings shift and take new forms for you, too.

Gratitudes

I labored over who and what to include in a gratitude list, because I cannot imagine leaving anything or anyone out. There have been such tiny, seemingly insignificant conversations that completely shifted my internal process or perspective. The amount of people, places and things that played a role in this is numberless and unknown.

I must offer this as gratitude to all the alignments known and unknown that have made me, and this, possible. Many bows to my spiritual team that guides me.

I want to say thank you to my many loves and all the forms they take. Especially my love Ollie, who has been in the thick of it with me. To my family, friends and loves in my life. You asked me how it was going, even when I did not want to talk about it, at all. Came over and did dishes for me. Prayed for me. Spoke ad nauseam with me about this project. Shared encouraging words, even when you were going through it yourself. Those of you who reminded me why I and this matters. Hung out with me in coffee shops for hours at a time. Stopped me when I was spiraling. Who sent me small gifts of support. Who let me know that you believed in what I was creating. Who laughed and hung out with me when I needed a break. For being generous with your views, that impacted mine. Recommended books or readings you thought I would be into (I was). Who saw this completed before I did. Listened to me read drafts aloud while cooking me a delicious meal. You who read drafts and offered feedback. Although I have not named you, I hope you see yourselves reflected here. To my loves, Kelli for the cover image and Alysha for all your contributions.

I owe so much of this to the many healing spaces that I have been lucky to encounter. Healers, diviners and teachers that focused on my body, my mind, my emotions and my spirit. My soulmate in healing, Cousin Nancie. To my many Sanghas and all the forms you take, thank you.

To one of my supervisors in particular Rebecca, who taught me "good enough," thank you. I want to thank the scholars and colleagues who told me to go for it. Who validated the urgency of this offering and it coming from my lens.

So much gratitude to my little sliver of the Atlantic Ocean in the Rockaways, to all the phases of the Moon, but the first quarter that I was born under that propels me. To the generosity of the Earth. To the lands of my ancestors, Ayiti and the land I am currently a guest of, Lenapehoking.

I need to offer gratitude to the people I have had the pleasure of serving. It is unfair how much I have received from you, how much you all have written this and I can only hope I have honored you well in these pages.

Chapter 1

Welcome To The Is-Ness

A Framework

Oppression is the bedrock of psychotherapy and the mental health and well-ness industries it resides in. Because these industries reinforce and replicate an oppressive society and culture. These industries are made up of people who were bred in or aspire to and have internalized the oppression of the culture. And due to this, most oppression goes unnoticed because they are acceptable social norms. They are even seen as moral or natural human behavior. Oppression comes from some fundamental beliefs that have evolved over time. In this book, we will explore those fundamental beliefs, their evolution and how they impact our work today.

The framework we will be using is based on my belief that for most of us, we have not had enough opportunity to really investigate why we believe the things we believe about the world, ourselves and each other. Through this investigation we will discover how many of our beliefs are actually inherited or we have been trained towards. Then, we pursue unlearning. We seek out where else there are beliefs to investigate. The pursuit leads us to seeing ourselves as a result rather than an individual equation. Seeing ourselves as a product of a bigger picture stirs up curiosity about what is possible if we reject being a product. It allows us to step out of the narrowness and rigidity oppression requires and notice what else is possible. It brings real choice. From this spacious place, we can hold that quality of space for people in our lives, whether clients or loved ones, including ourselves.

So let the unlearning begin. But first, some guidance.

Some Guidance

Ideally, I would be sitting in a circle with you and a few other people you care for and sharing the contents of this book with my voice. I could pause when I saw an expression that seemed confused or conflicted. We could have bio breaks and snack breaks. You could share out loud how the material is landing in you.

DOI: 10.4324/9781003207054-1

I would start us off in an embodied experience and use a voice that maintains the frequency of connectedness. We may laugh together a few times, and tears may come too. In an ideal world, I would be sitting with all the psychotherapists aspiring to take on an anti-oppressive practice in the West, just like that. The reality is, I cannot be in more than one place at once, nor do I want to be. So, I will offer some guidance on how to read this book that will bring a bit of the ideal world into the one we are currently in.

This book will always fall short of initiating all the arousal points in the mind and body that come alive when humans are in contact with other humans and other living things. It does not have the intelligence to receive expression or express itself in verbal or non-verbal communication. It will not be able to adjust to needs or find other ways to make an idea accessible. And for this reason, a book, although glorified, is terribly limited. There is so much these pages cannot say that could be simply shared in conversation or even a glance, and I am regretful of this and encouraged to try anyway. Writing this book is "within the degrees of contradiction that I have allowed myself."[1]

I recommend that you complete this book in community. With a few classmates, colleagues or friends. Commit to being in this together. This is different from a book club; this is not an academic endeavor, the invitation is to be in a practice group. Practice slowing down with each other and supporting each other to slow down. A group committed to staying present throughout. Gather a group of three to five people to read alongside you.

Word of Advice: do not join a mixed power group unless you already have an extensive practice around addressing power differentials and how they show up. If you have not already had this practice, I do not recommend reading together, even if you are in a preexisting reading group. Take time to develop and work on this important part of container building or bring in someone who can support and navigate what may arise in the group, not as a member, as a facilitator.

Engage in the collective as a space that wants to hear from each other. Make space to feel into what these ideas mean to you and how they land in your body. Ideally, you would begin your gatherings with some ritual that includes a collective grounding and end with a collective closing of the space. When I say grounding, I mean a practice that ushers more awareness to your body, a sense of connection to land/place, the group and self. In between the opening and ending, you read alongside each other; read a chapter at a time, discuss and share. Then have a meal together. This is no hour and a half Zoom meeting; this is network stitching. This is collective creation. I will speak to the importance of these types of connections in Part 3.

If you have picked up this book to read solo, it makes sense. We live in a very isolated culture and not many of us have connections that can hold us in our vulnerability. I hope there will be another opportunity for you to revisit this book with a collective in the near future.

We culturally have a tendency to only notice our bodies when there is an unpleasant sensation. The call to feel in this book is not only for where you feel an edge but where there is comfort and ease as well. The task of you as the reader is not to learn a lot of information or to memorize material; it is to let yourself feel impacted by what you are reading. What is coming up for you right now, knowing you will be asked to go slow? Is there resistance? Longing? Something else?

I hope you begin each chapter with a grounding. Let's do this first one together. I understand that what I am sharing may not be accessible for everyone. If you have a grounding practice of your own, use that one. If you hate this one, find one on the internet. Although I am going to do a body-centered grounding, you can do this by staring out to trees, playing a spacious piece of music that quiets your mind, by laying on grass, or by cuddling with a loved one or pet. What allows you to feel yourself, be present, curious, open, tender and receptive? That is what I hope you can drop into.

I will lead us now through this grounding exercise. Feel free to read it through first and then do what you remember on your own. This can take anywhere from 3 to 30 minutes, depending on your pacing. All of it is good. Do not time yourself; let yourself feel the instructions and how your body interprets them. Don't worry, you are doing it right.

Feel Into It

Still your body. Land in whatever posture requires the least amount of effort to maintain. Let the gaze of your eyes be soft or closed.

Take some deep breaths right here, right now.

Notice your body rising and falling to make space for the breath. Pay attention to the part of the body where you feel your breath the strongest and witness it.

Just noticing what expands with each inhale and what contracts with exhalation.

The brain will do what the brain does and jump ahead or look to analyze; just catch your mind when that happens and invite it back to notice your breath, without judgment.

Do a light scan of your body. If there are places that are activating for you, feel free to judgment-free skip. Take note of sensations without making meaning of them. Simply note and move on. If you want to release some tension- imagine/move some breath to that place when you inhale.

Notice your head. Forehead, face, back of your head.

Notice your torso, front, back, sides. Your shoulders, arms and hands and fingers. Notice your belly.

Notice your pelvis. Hips, groin, butt, genitals.

Notice your legs. Thighs front, back, sides. Knees, calves. Ankles and toes.

Notice when judgment or comparison happen and invite the mind back to the neutrality of noticing.

After your scan, return to noticing your breath.

Feel the space you are in. How each of your exhales impact the space, and with each inhale you take in the space. Consider the land of this space. How does that change the impact you want your breath to have and what you are taking in with each inhale?

Be with the invisible dance that is happening between you, your breath and everything around you. When you feel ready, prepare to open your eyes or focus your gaze. Feel into what you need to do that. Give yourself that and be slow to return fully outward.

Focus your gaze again, take in the space around you and notice what has your attention about your body, your emotions, your mind, your spirit.

Proceed to read with this inward attention present as much as you can. If it's hard or distracting, let it go, but commit to trying again later.

You did great! After you have grounded yourself, read as if you were listening. That might require reading the same line a few times; do that.

Notice how the words land on your personhood. If you are having a reaction, do not push past to finish. Stop, feel it, let it happen. Let it be big. Re-engage your grounding technique if you are not resourced enough to proceed into the bigness a feeling can take you to. I intend to impact you, the reader, so you have full permission from me to let it happen. I will also have some prompts as we go along, so if you do not naturally come to these pauses, there will be plenty of opportunities. Use those pauses as a moment to reflect as well. Feel free to record your reflections by writing, audio recording, drawing or movement. Share what feels most alive in you with your group.

My hope is that you let yourself be moved. This is the teaching. There are no definite truths in this offering because there are no definitive truths; your practice is what makes it true to you. Use all your senses to guide you through. There is no right way; your way is a good way.

My Apologies

Writing a book in the style of anti-oppression is hard and a big contradiction. I am still typing in the text of a language that has been forced on many cultures all over the globe. Still, here I am writing in this elitist method of communication that has been deemed as a superior while simultaneously made systemically and culturally inaccessible. My hope is that you, you the reader, can hear my voice while reading these pages. You can hear a real person speaking, at times, even ranting. This will not make it completely accessible, but it is worth the try.

When I think about writing a book, all I think about is how, by its nature, it aligns with oppression. When I use the word oppression, I mean any attachment to "truth" that disregards the truth of another. And so writing a book feels like something you do when you feel you know the truth and have a need to impart this truth on the still unknowing souls. As we will get into in later chapters, our attachment to knowing the "truth" is a symptom of neocortical supremacy and the precursor to oppression. In a capitalist society, we uphold facts as objective and trustworthy and feelings and experiences as subjective and fallible. In this society, we attach giving care to being worthy of care. A way to be deemed worthy of care is a perception of a person's ability and capacity to receive information, categorize it, recall that information, and utilize the information given. We are often asked to prove this in school, work and relationships. And in this culture, reading is like a loophole – signaling our worthiness to others.

A little history of reading may help us understand why it is seen as such a superior skill. During the Protestant Reformation in Western Europe, reading became a vital part of people saving their own souls. Newly converted protestants opened schools wherever they opened churches. These schools were primarily to teach everyone, including youth, how to read the Bible. The Reformation was a breakaway from the Catholic Church. They differed in that they believed that devotees should no longer rely on priests to interpret the Bible. Believers were expected to read the Bible themselves. This took their own salvation into their hands and secured their spot in heaven, but more importantly, guaranteed they wouldn't rot in hell.[2] This linked reading to redemption and virtuousness. And to this day, reading has maintained a sign of not only intelligence but virtue. Yet, reading has literally changed the structure of our brains, increasing our neocortical usage and conditioning us to be more analytical.[2]

Although not tied to religion directly anymore, reading in literate countries is riddled with its own judgments. Beginning in childhood, we encourage children to read in school. Giving them gold stars for knowing how to spell a word or for reading an extra paragraph at home after dinner. Children who enjoy reading are praised by adults and used as a comparison for other children who may struggle or simply dislike reading. The culture has equated the ability and desire to read as a superior intelligence. Reading somehow connotes that a person is using their brain more than others and, therefore, is a more valuable addition to society. And still there have been many systemic and cultural campaigns to keep groups of people from reading. For example, the Negro Act of 1740, a bill enacted in South Carolina, USA, made it punishable by law to teach an enslaved person to read or for an enslaved person to know how to read.[3] And more recently, the ongoing book bans happening across the country. Libraries, places for reading, are de-shelving books that relate people to each other, including those that explore race, gender, sexuality and other real variations of the human experience. There is a current continuous onslaught of legislation and legislators bringing back readings virtue signaling origins by banning books that illustrate the wide experiences of life on earth.

And so reading is a sign of virtue and a sign of superior intelligence reserved for those deemed as worthy. However, there are literally restrictions on who can read and what can be read. Those restrictions will not be considered when individual people are judged on their worthiness based on their ability to read. It is a virtue not everyone is actually expected to achieve yet can be punished for not possessing.

Our culture upholds that written facts (that change) are more reliable than the experiences of people, so storytelling, art, bodies, movement, senses are unreliable accounts of experience, while books are reliable and valuable accounts. And yet, books are edited often to correct misinformation. The data we think is irrefutable today will be disproven in a few years. In this book, I will attempt to observe a different wisdom – that the body's response to storytelling is a powerful way to express and share knowledge. That the emotions, the lessons elicited from storytelling, are more important than studies and data points that attempt to prove them.

Reading is an activity that is not inherently oppressive. It is a mode of communication. What has become oppressive is that we uplift it as a superior and primary way to express, learn and communicate, which, in turn, has suppressed, shamed and made invalid the many ways beings can share knowledge.

My deepest apologies for using this medium to offer what I have accumulated; however, as we continue to learn together, I will disclose many ways I am still indoctrinated in oppression and it is my continued work to liberate myself and others while being honest about my contradictions. What I do not want to do is what academics do to protect their egos, as described by Alice Miller, "[S]ome professors or writers who are quite capable of expressing themselves clearly will use language that is so convoluted and arcane that their students or readers must struggle angrily to acquire ideas that they can make little use of."[4] I have been that reader, and hope that at no point you are that reader here.

You will see I do not quote many studies because, to this day, 90 percent of the participants in psychological research and studies are college students of the West or university students of other nations that were required to take on Western ideals of analytics to be in university.[2] That means many of these studies that are supposed to inform us on "human nature" are done with people who have adapted to Western psychology. Therefore, the studies only validate themselves.

Another apology I must make is that I will be clumping Western society together in this book. I am sorry for the ways that erase other cultures that are within this society. I am not ignoring the millions of bodies, minds, hearts that do not benefit from this society and are oppressed within it. I am spotlighting the dominant culture we are forcibly made to navigate. I will speak to other ways of being, lightly, not to compare or to say they are better or we should steal from them (American reflex) but to expand possibilities. I am sorry to all the cultures, societies and histories that will not be realized in these pages.

I will not really separate out white cis-men even though I know that they are the perpetrators of a lot of what I will be naming in the book. I am not splitting up Westerners because even I play into it. Audre Lorde reminds me that "it is easier to deal with the external manifestations" of these systems "than it is to deal with the results of those distortions internalized within our consciousness of ourselves and one another."[5] Even now, so many of us who are shoved into the margins, who are not the intended audience of these norms, and are actually the bodies othered to normalize white cis-men's beliefs of their superiority, have found our way to whiteness, and cis, white male power through our submission to neocortical supremacy and the performance of that through our professions. I will speak specifically to the profession of psychotherapy. And so, although I will not be naming or speaking to white supremacy directly, it is simply because I am looking at how we have internalized these ideals to get a little piece of the pie. And that's actually what I want us to tackle, not really looking at anyone else. I'm asking us to look at ourselves.

An Origin Story

As a child, I wanted to be a psychologist. Fleeting visions of me sitting on my throne, sitting back while the weak and hopeless spilled unto me their problems so I can help fix them. And somewhere in life, those visions went away. I began aligning myself more with the person spilling out. I would have been seen as depressed if I were enrolled in counseling as a young person. Home, everyday after school for hours, laying on the couch. Not wanting to die, but not quite attached to living. Feeling so alone, and responsible for my loneliness. I was a Black bi-cultural, sexually confused, fat girl born of immigrant parents in a big city of the United States. Everything about me was supposed to feel shameful. As Sonya Renee Taylor writes in *The Body is Not an Apology*, the colonized culture makes certain bodies more shameful than others.[6] And I did. I did feel ashamed and lonely.

In fact, although I had dreams of becoming a therapist, it took me years of walking in front of the psychologist office before I had the courage to go in. What I wanted most and what I feared was that I would walk in and fall apart. Instead of letting that happen, I got strong. I contained my feelings, I became funnier and sharper – much better skills to have in my environment. I disconnected further from my shameful body and became more neocortically dependent. I did what I needed to do to stay under the radar – and shied away from any spaces where my deficiencies could be seen.

I went to college and joined every organization available. I became a student organizer and activist. I was overwhelmed in the ways the world was wrong and I was consumed with changing that. I joined and led students to action in an attempt to take power away from powerful people. I was becoming powerful. That power had to go somewhere, and why shouldn't it be me? I locked my sights on becoming a policymaker, to work in legislation. I had crafted this personality where people trusted me; they knew I would deliver. It became easy for me to maneuver a world where I was liked, respected and trusted – therefore, I knew I could always have access to power. Being lonely was acceptable, but the feeling of powerlessness became unbearable. I was living this fear that I could not "grow beyond whatever distortions" I would find in myself, so I focused on being "externally defined."[7]

When exploring politics, I was continually heartbroken by how quickly politicians lost their luster, fast. So, I thought, "Clearly, they were all raised poorly; I will help children." I went to work with young people, then I realized they have very little power in their lives, "I need to work with parents." I started working with parents on parenting (although I had no children), teaching "evidence-based" parenting models. Then I realized these parents cannot do the techniques because they are riddled with trauma, "I must help the adults who go on to have children." So, I found myself doing clinical work in a non-profit. I still call myself a reluctant therapist, although I have actually returned to what I knew about myself before I shut down that quality of knowing.

Simultaneously with my new career as a clinical therapist, Black Lives Matter (BLM) influenced the social conversations happening and usage of media. Social media became a tool to inform, and with this tool, I found so many reasons to hate the world. My understanding of capitalism and colonization and their impacts increased. I became well-versed in the ways oppression had shown black indigenous and people of color that we were inferior beings. Oppression was a survival technique that those aligned with white supremacy were using to avoid extinction, an extinction that Black people and colonized people all over the world know too well.

James Baldwin said, "To be a Negro in this country and to be relatively conscious is to be in a rage almost all the time."[8] That could not be more true for this period in my life. I was enraged. But more than enraged, I was hopeless. And I was ashamed of feeling hopeless. It felt taboo to admit to myself or anyone else. On top of my work as a therapist, I was found regularly at a protest, direct action, a lecture, an organizing meeting. I leaned into my rage, which led me to more ways to get involved. It was never enough. I was jumping on whatever actions came across my newsfeed (and there were plenty), signed whatever petition was circulating, depending on my cash flow, donated to whatever cause seemed urgent enough, I shared articles as a tool of awareness. I was at all the talks, lectures and workshops trying to learn more about this beast we were living in, soaking up the strategies people were building and finding ways to adopt them all. Like Audre Lorde, "[M]y anger has meant pain to me but it has also meant survival, and before I give it up I'm going to be sure that there is something at least as powerful to replace it."[9] I was looking everywhere for that powerful replacement.

But what I felt under the anger was not more powerful, it was hopelessness, which in these spaces translated to weakness. I could not really say aloud I felt hopeless. It felt like a betrayal. It was condescending to the struggle. It was like erasing the work that so many others have done. My secret hopelessness increased my longtime isolation. And to avoid that, I did more. My understanding was that if I were actively organizing, I'd feel less hopeless; if I were doing work I believed in, I'd feel less hopeless. Instead, isolation and despair began to eat away at me. The rage was all I could express that was safe, so it was all I allowed myself to see.

While trying to manage my rage against the world and secret hopelessness, I was a decent therapist. Seemingly, working with folks to recognize and challenge their beliefs, increasing insight about major "malfunctioning" parts of their identities or behaviors. I created a lot of treatment plans focusing on modifying behaviors, from small and unnoticeable adjustments to large and drastic modifications that would cause chaos in their lives outside of the counseling room but earned clients praise in it. The changes were much scarier done than said, so we talked about them a lot, making them great service goals! That was decent counseling. Work done under the conditions of capitalism "robs our work of its erotic value, its erotic power and life appeal and fulfillment."[7]

Decent counseling is not directly harmful, but it ensures distance between myself and the other. And to be distant from the other, I needed to maintain distance from myself, my instincts, feelings and senses. Distance that was solidified in me in graduate school. Distance that is hailed as a healthy part of the therapeutic relationship in many therapeutic modalities. Distance that would withstand any ethics check. A distance unremarkable to discuss or to be noticed, until it was so loud it could not be ignored.

An Undesirable Choice Point

I had a brilliant client, let's call them RL. When I say brilliant, I do not mean intelligent, although they were that as well, I mean radiant. I mean their presence illuminated space; they freely emanated warmth. RL was one of my first psychotherapy clients. RL was a Black queer person who just entered their seventh decade on the planet when we met. RL had a longtime companion and intimate co-dependent relationship with Heroin. RL had been with heroin since they were a late teenager after the death of their mother. RL came out to their seemingly healthy mother as a queer person a week prior to their mother's death and blamed themselves for her heart malfunction. They believed that they made her heart weak. And after everyone moved on from helping them grieve, RL had Heroin. For four decades RL fought with heroin. Heroin was the villain and the savior of their life. I was so drawn to RL. They reminded me of an elder I have never had. They were hilarious and curt, they were honest and reflective, they were hurt and childlike.

We had a fabulous relationship. They seemed to see me as a cross between a close friend and a magical child. I had so many urges to lean all the way into RL and their "projections." I wanted to play fully into the role of the magical child or the good friend. I wanted to be liked by them, but through my education and supervision I knew that would be inappropriate. I struggled to do as I was trained, to steer away from the human connection that was strongly present between us. I worked harder to manage myself and maintain appropriate distance.

RL was passively suicidal. Never attempted suicide while working with me, but looked for relief in heroin that often led them to take heroic doses, or risky combinations with heroin. They came in with stories that made me fear for their life and experiences that made me want to hold them dearly. Yet, I did none of the above. And because I learned my fear was irrelevant and needed to be managed, I did not invite them to feel into their fear either.

The beginning of our relationship, I worked hard to do as I was taught, help them understand why they were "abusing drugs" so they could become normal. Normal meaning that they stop needing drugs and replace them with a more acceptable addiction like earning money or romantic entanglements. After some time, I considered that this method did not feel like it was in their best interest. They lived in insecure housing, they had no other intimate relationships and they were an elder in a world that despised aging. I started questioning if sobriety would be more supportive than Heroin in keeping them on the planet. I decided to move away from the script and we began working on them forgiving heroin instead. We started working on trying to understand why they hated Heroin, when it seems to be so good to them. Most of this exploration never ended up about Heroin itself. It went back to people who abandoned them because of their relationship to Heroin. It came back to that Heroin made them act and behave in ways that were unacceptable and brought them much rejection in life. It was about the people that Heroin seemed to encourage to abandon RL. At the same time, Heroin helped them deal with all the rejection and loneliness. We started working on seeing Heroin as an ally in a difficult world. A companion that was doing its best to be there for them but sometimes did more than it was suited for. This intervention, accepting the relationship was harder for RL than taking on blame and responsibility for their addiction, which they already were so familiar with as they have been in abstinence-based rehab many times.

Soon after this pivot and months into seeing RL, who never missed a session without alerting me, they "no called, no showed." The following week, as we were approaching what would have been their next appointment, someone who lived in their building who knew they were getting counseling at the agency called and informed us that RL died. I learned that they died from a fall, I assumed, while with Heroin.

Initially, I was shocked. And I cannot recall grief and sadness, but I am sure they were there. What I remember, what I will never forget, was the rage. When I write this right now, when I think of them or speak of them (which I do often), there are tears; what accompanies the tears is a heat that radiates all over my body on my skin. I can see myself turning into fire. At that time, that fire consumed me because that rage had been boiling up in me for some time and it was ready for this moment.

First, there was rage towards the world. How could someone live most of their life in the wars of their own mind and that be alright with society? How could someone live their whole life alone in this world? What kind of culture found it acceptable that there were millions of people who lived lives in isolation like RL? Then came the rage towards myself. How could I be so cold and distant? I could feel their suffering. What was I so afraid of? Why didn't I dive all the way in? Why was I so scared to be human with another human? Then, rage towards my profession. What are we doing exactly? Are we training to be placeholders for a good life? Where is the humanity in this field? This was when I began investigating the role of Social Work, Mental Health Industry and oppression.

Through my explorations, I came to read *Radical Dharma: Talking Race, Love, And Liberation* by Rev. angel Kyodo williams, Lama Rod Owens and Jasmine Syedullah. This book pointed me towards what was under all that rage; there, I found that old hopelessness again. I couldn't ignore it or push it away this time. It consumed me.

Here was my choice point. Would I continue to push away this heartbreak and hopelessness in exchange for false optimism or a hollow belief in change or would I finally let the hopelessness be real, and be full? I leaned all the way into it and it led to nowhere else but more rage, more hopelessness and a circling of the two. Until my first guided psychedelic experience, where what came through strongly was grief. So much grief about the impossibility of these times, but also all the grief of my ancestors, of Black people who have died at the hands of oppression and its agents. The grief and hopelessness that my good intentions meant nothing in a society that only dishes suffering. What I grieved most was how much of this I had been hiding from myself. In the grief, I always encountered that I had dreams, I had wishes, there was possibility. "And to acknowledge our dreams is to sometimes acknowledge the distance between those dreams and our present situation."[5] That is being in the is-ness, the present, what is true.

This process, that is ongoing, transformed my life, transformed my worldview, transformed my practice. The grief and heartbreak I keep close to me now is a compass towards what is actually here and then to what is possible. Going towards my heartbreak brings me to the erotic power Audre Lorde writes of, which I think of as limbic connection. The erotic is clear, "the dichotomy between the spiritual and the political is also false."[7] It opens up to all the unseen connections that I ignore to stay neocortical and in control. It directs me towards my next movements as much as it directs me to stop moving. It makes space in me to be receptive to others and their grief and pain and to seek it out rather than turn away. It brings me a quiet and accepting spirit. It brings me my longing for connection. It invites me to inhabit the is-ness. It breaks me out of illusion. This society requires illusion to stay afloat.

Diagnosing a Society

I mean this society is psychopathic. I am choicefully using that word. This culture would easily meet criteria for an official DSM Antisocial Personality diagnosis. Some criteria to meet this diagnosis include:[10]

- It uses deceitfulness, as indicated by repeated lying, use of aliases, or conning others for personal profit or pleasure.
- It contains much irritability and aggressiveness, as indicated by repeated physical fights or assaults.
- It has a reckless disregard for the safety of self or others.
- And most importantly, lack of remorse, as indicated by being indifferent to or rationalizing having hurt, mistreated, or stolen from another.

Let's take a breather here; there are some American sociopathic examples ahead. If you are resourced enough, please read it; if you are not, please take a break and then read. However you do it, turning away from truth is the opposite of the ask I am making of you.

At this point (late 2022), the US has let 1.09 million people die of COVID-19.[11] These are reported COVID-19-related deaths, and yet all of their policy and communication denies science and data that recommends stopping business as usual to stop this death count. Instead, the country pretends that 1.09 million people are not missing from it and encourages everyone to go shopping again, go out to eat to restimulate the economy and go back to normal.[12]

As of late 2022, there are recorded 622 mass shootings or mass murders in the US since 2013.[13] To remedy this, we have children do shooting drills in school where they pretend a person with a gun has entered the school and they must find good places to hide.[14] We debate giving teachers guns, add more blood-thirsty police in schools and see owning assault rifles as freedom.[15]

Speaking of children, in 2019, Black birthing parents were 243 percent more likely than white birthing parents to die of "pregnancy related causes,"[16] while we have politicians campaigning that the US maternal mortality rate is not too bad, if you do not count Black people.[17] This campaign to not see Black people as human is the same ideology that is used in all colonization efforts. If some people are not human, then we do not need to care for or protect them.

A small taste of how this cruelty has impacted other parts of the world. Monsanto made India into a big laboratory for their products, making farmers completely reliant on their expensive and toxic products that were not outfitted for the climate. This has impoverished many farmers, devastating the industry and the people who make it up. Unable to make a living, by 2013, about 250,000 farmers committed suicide in the 16 years prior, "making it the largest wave of recorded suicides in human history."[18]

And just to add some historical sociopathic behavior, in the 1800s, white Americans ate Black people. White people boiled and ate Nat Turner.[19] This became a heated debate and discourse of the time. I hope this registered that they had to discuss whether or not they should keep allowing it to happen, fearing they would *appear* cannibalistic.

I know I am using the DSM to justify my rant here, but the field of psychology is sociopathic itself. Including the former mental illness "drapetomania," which was the illness that enslaved people would be diagnosed with if they tried to run away.[20] The prescribed treatment for this condition was cruel and I will not describe it here.

I share all this because I do not think we all need such personally painful choice points as I experienced with RL's death. This book is an offering of a choice point. A choice point where you get to decide whether you want to go along with psychotherapy in a sociopathic society or if you want to feel the goodness of your heart and the impossibility of this work in this world and grieve it. And let that grief be the rich soil for something else. I obviously am biased towards the latter, but either way, this is your choice. The value of RL's life was not for my awakening, but I am grateful to have the value of mine increased by knowing them. And through this transmission, I hope you can say the same.

Why Now?

All of that is my why now?

Be present to your own questions as to why you picked up this offering. Why now? What has brought you here? What are the questions you are asking of yourself and others that landed you to look at your work as political, healing or justice-oriented? What deep, quiet part of you has driven you all these years? What does it hope to find in these pages? These questions, along with your breath, will be your anchors.

There is our personal "why this book" and "why now," but there is also a social "why" that makes engaging in this work timely. This work is the work of investigating what our roles are in the mental health field; reflecting on our individual and personal investments in the oppression that the mental health industry rests on, and committing to being a witness and interrupter of oppression in ourselves and others.

Oppression is being unveiled everywhere. Not to be confused with it has never existed. Collectively around the globe, the impacts of oppression and ongoing demonstration of more oppression are taking center stage. We can no longer hide from the histories and ongoing consequences of colonization. We are being confronted with how we engage in oppression even when we are unaware. Space is being made for the consequences to be named in personal relationships, in institutions and in social norms.

At the same time, we are seeing capitalism and colonialism double down to preserve power in overt and subtle ways. People are awakening to their roles in maintaining the status quo. And without seeing our personal investments in oppression, even as we reject those ideals, we will collude with them.

It is an overwhelming time. For many, they continue to ignore the suffering they have caused or been accomplice to, but for some, the awareness of their role in social contracts has become devastating. This may lead to some paralysis of what are the right changes to make towards reducing oppression or at least doing less oppressing themselves. And the advice is never-ending. Every day, new books to read, listicles sharing "the best ways to be an ally to . . .", social media posts, images, long texts with considerations for shift in language, shift in how to behave, shift in how to interact with others. And it changes based on context, relationships and time. It is a lot.

This book is an invitation for clinicians to not succumb to the paralysis of political correctness, but to connect deeply to our personal relationships to oppression and the pain and suffering we experience. Then to use that connection to help us navigate social and professional interactions. Allowing the intelligence that emerges from this exploration to help us slow down, be reflective and vulnerable; connect to other humans and living things, granting us the spaciousness to hold complexity in support of us responding in a way that does not look away from oppression and informs us on how we can cause the least amount of harm in the moment. This time is not for neocortical intelligence; it is not brilliant enough for this task; this is a time for limbic intelligence. This is not easy; it is barely capturable in that sentence. This process, this commitment is years and years of work. And it should take that long. It took you (your current age) and a few generations before you to become who you are at this moment. If you intend to change in a few months, you are not being reasonable or kind to yourself or your history. And so, if one individual life will take years to undo some small but important aspect of their life, imagine the case for a culture, for a society. It took us centuries to develop the current social contracts we are steeped in. Imanuel Wallerstein offered to a group of people I was lucky to be part of at the USSF 2010 an important reminder that our society is changing, that is inevitable; to interrupt the direction it is going, it is about sowing seeds. I have taken this to heart – let every interaction I am in be a sowing of a seed. And I have some bigger idealistic seeds as well.

Idealistically, if people no longer saw their worth tied to oppression, if they were able to return to their body as the holder of information and their truths, if they turned to human connection, connection to lineage, land, other non-human beings as their desired mode of survival, life as we know it would have to change. Families, communities, leadership, power would have to change. Fortunately, Mental Health practitioners are at the perfect location to support someone to do that work. We are in the right position to guide our clients into loosening the relationship between their innate worth and their own oppression. We can encourage reconnecting bodies to minds to spirits. We get to witness the leaps into desirable connections with self and others. We can explore with them what is possible; if there is nowhere else in their lives to imagine, they can with us. However, to do that work, we must take on this work for ourselves.

Sonya Renee Taylor writes, "We struggle to hold the truths of others because we have so rarely had the experience of having our truths held."[6] You cannot teach, share, give something you do not have. The work we do with the people we serve is a direct reflection of how we perceive ourselves, and our location in the world. If we want people to expand past what they know to be possible, we need to seek the impossible as well. We need to feel the satisfaction of looking back and realizing we have already seen impossible, and so there are more impossibles to come. We need to believe we are, in us and around us, a whole world of possibilities that have not been met yet. This is another angle of the erotic – "it is an internal sense of satisfaction to which, once we have experienced it. We know we can aspire."[7] It becomes our compass.

Lorde goes on to declare that this satisfaction compels us to make connections where we can share our joys rather than using others as objects of satisfaction.[7] This leads us to reward interdependence rather than individualistic, analytical and "power over" behaviors. As someone bred in the Mental Health field, I know the inclination is to reward our clients for building relationships in their lives, but the invitation I am making here is to be in an interdependent relationship with each other, you and them. The ask is simple yet incredibly difficult: what would it look like to de-professionalize our work and reclaim its erotic power? And are you willing to do what it takes?

So, What's Next?

This book aims to move you, the therapist, through a complicated intervention. This intervention is a practice. "It is a practice of shifting the way we pay attention, the way our body responds to new information."[21] The practice is geared towards being in liberated communities and the anti-oppressive stance we as clinicians must take to join them. Anti-oppression is about widening our view.

The practice is broken into three major categories. These categories will guide this book. They are:

1. We must interrupt neocortical supremacy in ourselves.
   Part 1 will be all about reminding us that whatever we know, is made up. Neocortical supremacy is the belief that because of the size of our frontal lobe, we are superior to all other beings on the planet, that we have the right to dominate them, that we are the top of the food chain. Neocortical supremacy believes that because we use it to strategize, categorize and take action it is the most important part of being a human. That it is the entirety of what we should rely on to understand ourselves, others and the worlds we are part of. Finally, neocortical supremacy believes and makes it true that those who have abandoned all the other ways of being on the planet/world for itself are more

civilized than others. This warped, unnatural logic has led to and justified the demonization and terrorization of the world. We have to recognize we are more than our neocortex. This pulling the ground from underneath makes our habits clear, brings attention to the ways we function without deep consideration. When we divest from the neocortex being the only way to make sense of things, we search for other ways of knowing. This leads us to Part 2.

2. We must engage our limbic system.

    What happened to the other ways of knowing? How have we been disconnected from them? Part 2 is all about us as Western-trained and oriented clinicians. How we have been taught to ignore our bodies. Our bodies are our limbic messengers. The severing of this connection keeps us in our neocortex and away from all that we do not understand, that we do not yet know, that is not habit, that is choice. Keeps us from the unseen and unknowable and from being nature. We explore how we have been enrolled into maintaining this disconnection. Part 2 is a reminder that what we seek is in us already and it is informed, influenced and responsive to the same structures that buried it. "We begin to discern what is ours and what is not ours."[21]

3. Limbic resonance needs other beings.

    Part 3 is about the importance of moving this practice out of the individual and into the collective. Neocortical supremacy has continually robbed us of belonging, while the limbic system needs it. Here, we will discuss the importance of reconnecting with the other and how to bring this perspective to clients.

Feel Into It

Hey! This is your first prompt! Whenever you come across these, feel encouraged to pause. You are invited to use these prompts to feel something in you. You are also invited to record your responses to share with your reading group. Here we go!

Pick a location that you can feel on your body. Does not matter what part as long as you can actually feel it. Internal sense or external touch. And take a few moments here, learning about it. What is happening there?

How intense is it?

Does it come with a sense of color? Temperature? Texture? Sensation?

Does it change as you remain attentive to it?

Return to this place when and where you can as you continue reading.

Practice to Intervention

I utilize activities like this when someone does not believe they can feel their body and are trapped in making-sense-land. Sometimes, I have to bring attention to a part. Like "I see your hands are gripping each other, how does that feel?" or "Do you feel your feet on the ground? That is part of your body." In a culture where if we do not "know for sure" it does not exist, activities as simple as this help someone to feel into small openings of information they are not considering or seeing as valid.

Once you have done this exercise yourself, consider:

- How do you think a focal point activity like this can be beneficial to some of your clients?
- Which ones?
- When would it make sense to engage in an activity like this?

Citations

1. Joseph, G. (1995). Black feminist pedagogy and schooling in capitalist White America. In B. Guy-Sheftall (Ed.), *Words of fire: An anthology of African American feminist thought*. The New Press.
2. Henrich, J. (2021). *WEIRDest people in the world: How the west became psychologically peculiar and particularly prosperous*. Picador Paper.
3. The Equal Justice Initiative. (n.d.). *May 10, 1740 | South Carolina passes negro act of 1740, codifying White supremacy*. https://calendar.eji.org/racial-injustice/may/10
4. Miller, A. (1997). *The drama of the gifted child: The search for the true self* (revised ed., 3rd ed.). Basic Books.
5. Lorde, A. (2007). Eye to eye: Black women, hatred, and anger. In *Sister outsider*. The Crossing Press. (Original work published 1983)
6. Taylor, S. R. (2018). *The body is not an apology: The power of radical self-love* (16pt large print ed.) (Large type/Large print). ReadHowYouWant.
7. Lorde, A. (2019). Uses of the erotic: The erotic as power. In A. M. Brown (Ed.), *Pleasure activism: The politics of feeling good*. AK Press. (Original work published 1984)
8. NPR. (2020, June 1). To be in a rage, almost all the time. *NPR.org*. www.npr.org/2020/06/01/867153918/-to-be-in-a-rage-almost-all-the-time
9. Lorde, A. (2007). The uses of anger: Women responding to racism. In *Sister outsider*. The Crossing Press. (Original work published 1983)
10. Psychiatric News. (2004). *DSM-IV-TR* Diagnostic criteria for antisocial personality disorder (301.7). *Psychiatric News*, *39*(1), 25–25. https://doi.org/10.1176/pn.39.1.0025a
11. Tracking Covid-19's global spread. (n.d.). *CNN*. https://edition.cnn.com/interactive/2020/health/coronavirus-maps-and-cases/
12. Peralta, J. (2020, November 30). *Here's how to stimulate the global economy in a climate-protective way*. The Rockefeller Foundation. www.rockefellerfoundation.org/blog/heres-how-to-stimulate-the-global-economy-in-a-climate-protective-way/
13. *Gun violence archive*. (n.d.). www.gunviolencearchive.org/
14. Blad, E. (2022, June 9). School shooter drills: Is there a right way to do them? *Education Week*. www.edweek.org/leadership/school-shooter-drills-is-there-a-right-way-to-do-them/2022/06
15. Mervosh, S. (2022, August 5). After Uvalde, a kindergarten teacher trains to carry a gun in school. *The New York Times*. www.nytimes.com/2022/07/31/us/teachers-guns-schools.html

16. Winters, M. (2020). *Black fatigue: How racism erodes the mind, body, and spirit* (Illustrated). Berrett-Koehler Publishers.
17. Levin, B. (2022, May 21). *Louisiana senator bill Cassidy: Our maternal death rates are only bad if you count black women.* Vanity Fair. www.vanityfair.com/news/2022/05/bill-cassidy-maternal-mortality-rates
18. Thanissara. (2015). *Time to stand up: An engaged Buddhist manifesto for our earth -- The Buddha's life and message through feminine eyes (sacred activism)* (1st ed.). North Atlantic Books.
19. Kat, S. A. (2021). *Postcolonial astrology: Reading the planets through capital, power, and labor.* North Atlantic Books.
20. Harrison, D. L., & Laymon, K. (2021). *Belly of the beast: The politics of anti-fatness as anti-blackness.* North Atlantic Books.
21. Leiner, R., & Syedullah, J. (2023). The manual for liberating survival: Lesson I, how self-care matters as an embodied practice of abolition. In A. Crawley & R. Sirvent (Eds.), *Spirituality and abolition.* Common Notions.

Part 1

Disrupting Neocortical Supremacy

Chapter 2

Historical Context

Widening Our View

To understand anti-oppression truly, we need to expand past the initially easier route, which is to blame some mean people. To truly be anti-oppressive, we need to be willing to see how the very assumptions we make about how humans are oppressive. Oppression is not a set of actions; it is a belief system. It is a belief system that undergirds Western psychology, institutions and relationships. Oppression invades every aspect of Western life; it has destructively impacted the entire world. This chapter explores the assumptions we have come to accept as human nature that are oppressive.

Feel Into It

Here, we are going to challenge the neocortex by exploring some assumptions. This exploration may feel challenging to our neocortex, which has already neatly categorized some of it as universally true due to the cultural reinforcement of these assumptions. There might even be some chaos in your system based on some of these explorations. Notice that.

What are the signs that you are resistant to new information in your body? If you don't already know them, pay attention. Check in on your jaw, shoulders and hips.

Practice to Intervention

Chaotic energy can be very alarming. For myself, I tend to feel nauseous, like I cannot catch my thoughts, sometimes even my breath; like I am having an internal battle but cannot distinguish the sides from each other. I speak less, stutter more and often can feel anguish on my face.

For one client, I know we have hit chaos because they get very combative with me. Something that has come up does not align with the narrative

DOI: 10.4324/9781003207054-3

they have of themselves or the world and they cannot take it in. They sit upright, like a judge and begin to push away anything said. In these moments, I have to recognize the chaos happening and name "Something's changed. What's happening right now?" Sometimes, due to our relationship, they may reflect on it next session and say something like, "I did not like that, but I've sat with it and there is something to that; can we explore that?"

After spending time learning about how your system recognizes chaos, pay attention to your clients. What does chaos, confusion do to them? What are the signs that they are in territory that is difficult? How do you bring attention to those signs? How do you honor and not override those?

For me, Unlearning is mostly about increasing what is possible by getting very comfortable with how much we have deemed as impossible. Because "experience methodically rewires the brain, and the nature of what it has seen dictates what it can see."[1] In other words, you see only what you can already imagine. Although this may be true of all human brains, it is especially true of the Western brain, which over-relies and over-uses the neocortex since we actually only scan for "useful" information. Scanning for information we expect to be useful already lends itself to staying within our range of possibility. This limits what information we take in and makes our view narrow.

For example, in a study identifying facial emotions across cultures, researchers placed various images of a group of people in front of Japanese and American participants, with one person in the front of the pack; let's call them Kris. The participants were asked to describe how Kris felt based on the image. Americans never took their eyes off of Kris to explain how they felt, while the Japanese people did a lot of scanning and their responses would change based on the expressions of the other people behind Kris.[2] Americans don't take their eyes off the target. That is because Westerners have an analytic dominant view. Our culture is deeply reliant on a narrow lens so we can better analyze and take action towards the target rather than see the entirety of the scene. This analysis, calculation and categorization primarily happens in the neocortex.

But to be an anti-oppressive clinician, we must shatter that narrow lens. Adolf Guggenbuhl-Craig encourages that "the psychotherapist must be challenged by something which cannot be either mastered or fended off by his analytical weapons and techniques."[3] Taking on these challenges allows our view to be broader. That's what this anti-oppressive thing is about. If we only use the fields of social science and psychology to understand our work and the people we work with, we are remaining narrowly focused. In this chapter, we will look at material that usually resides in the camps of anthropology, politics, history, philosophy and economics to help fill out our holistic view. These actually have been split apart with time from each other as our psychologies in the West became more and more focused and specialist-oriented.[4] By seeking to bring together these specialties, we attempt to have a holistic view.

Anti-oppressive clinicians are holistic perceivers.

Holistic thinkers focus not on the parts but on the whole, and specifically on the relationships between the parts or on how they fit together. And as part of a larger web of complex relationships, they expect time trends to be nonlinear or even cyclical by default.[5]

So, if being holistic is an option, how did we end up here in analytical land? My aim is to create a trail to answer just that. How did we become collectively analytical and a culture fixated on our target, ignoring the rest? To dive into this, we will be going on a generally linear but cyclical journey through the creation of the analytic individual. To begin, we need to actually build a fundamental understanding of our current society. A deep dive that honors that cultures evolve, not through spontaneous combustion, but through the right conditions and collective consciousness. Henrich writes, "[Y]ou can't truly understand psychology without considering how the minds of populations have been shaped by cultural evolution."[5] In this field and in our culture, we believe that our psychologies are individual and, at the same time, we believe there is a normal psychology to aspire towards. Studying cultural evolution enlists a curiosity about how normal psychologies came to be and how does that impact me, a client, a loved one, the individual?

An anti-oppressive seat is about just that, developing a curiosity about the historical underpinnings that have brought "us" to where we are today. There are so many histories worth sharing and telling, and this one is not superior by any means, but it is the most relevant to understanding our current psychology. When I say "our" or "us" I mean what Henrich and colleagues coined W.E.I.R.D people. This acronym stands for societies that are Western, Educated, Industrialized, Rich and Democratic.[5]

Cultural Evolution, Not Social Darwinism

Before we move on, let's clarify cultural evolution. As clinicians, we are taught to cling to Darwinian evolution, but we are not encouraged to study cultural evolution. Social Darwinism is the belief that the more dominant survive and the weak deserve termination. But actually, most of human evolution in the last 20,000 years came about as unconscious overlapping combinations of rituals, social norms and taboos, not genetic superiority.[5] The ongoing combinations that build on one another is cultural evolution.

Social Darwinism (survival of the fittest) is about superiority, while Darwinism itself is about observing change. Cultural evolution is about changes in societies that are influenced by land, collective consciousness and adaptation.

Social Darwinism actually does little to explain why we do things. "While we have a certain biological makeup, we are not genetically programmed to feel or believe or act in any particular manner."[6] The culture someone is adapted in can and does override genetic tendencies.[1]

This is important to begin with because this belief that some genes are better suited to survive shows up in much of what we consider "natural." Clinging to genetic evolution and social Darwinism allows us to shed responsibility. We can chalk things up to "the natural order of things." Or language we use in our field, like "predisposition," meaning that a person's suffering could have been predicted based on their genetics. This means we do not have to look at the conditions that are cultural, structural, economic, political and environmental that have also contributed. Not taking away that genetics has an impact; they just explain a lot less than we give them credit for.

For example, today, Black people are least likely in the West to be taken seriously about medical or emotional distress due to us being "predisposed" to things like hypertension, diabetes and aggression. But we also know about allostatic load, which is the measurable accumulation of stress in the body that impacts genetic imprints and bodily functions, such as hormone production and metabolism. We also know that allostatic load increases with ongoing experiences of threats like discrimination and the stress of work. We know about the vagus nerve, the system of nerves that translate senses into information for our nervous system.[7] We also know that when under constant threat, animals, including humans, can fight or flight, which is orchestrated by the vagal nervous system. Threats can look like discrimination or threats to livelihood through work. So with all of these that we know, it is common to hear practitioners of different disciplines explain away Black people's complaints because of disposition instead of looking at the context that is causing the physical, emotional and spiritual body to respond the way it is. That's using the belief that some beings are not fit to survive and, therefore, may not be worth the effort of helping. That is social Darwinism at play.

But cultural evolution shifts that responsibility back to us. Having a curiosity about cultural evolution discourages this dismissal and encourages us to expand our attention and see a person as part of a much bigger picture. To embrace their suffering as more complicated than their genetics.

So, let's shift our attention towards history so we can learn more about some of the pieces we can take into account.

Feel Into It:

We are about to go into a bunch of history; what do you need to stay present and allow yourself to be impacted? Take a moment. Get what you need. We'll wait.

Now that you have what you need. Note again that some of this can be challenging or validating; allow yourself to let information sink in. If you find something evoking a particularly strong sense, take a break and let it happen. Record what feels comforting to read, what in your body indicates comfort, what makes you anxious or agitated to read; how do you know in your body; where are you neutral; how does neutral present?

Practice to Intervention

Neutral is a feeling. It has components to it. Really learn your neutral. What habits or automatic actions happen in this state? Those are worth studying.

With clients, we can do a lot by bringing attention to their neutral stance. Start paying attention. Do not just pay attention for yourself. How do you share your observations so your observations can be confirmed, challenged, tweaked?

Let's Start From Somewhere Towards the End

Our human ancestors have been roaming the planet for, what seems to me, an inconceivable amount of time. We will start towards the end. Even when our (here I mean human) ancestors were nomadic roamers, they were in competition, like every other species on the planet. Not competition as in sport, or aggression. Competition as in creating the best combination of rituals, taboos and norms to survive.

"Humanity began in a precarious world where tiny bands foraged and scrimped for food by day, huddled together for warmth by night."[1] This may sound reminiscent of a camp excursion and a cute campfire at night; this is not that. It was viciously cold and this was necessary to survive the cold of the planet at the time. At that time, the Earth was cooler, and with low CO_2 levels, manipulating the land was not possible. These nomads engaged in what we now call hunter-gatherer societies.

Hunter-gatherers who were in largely spread-out networks thrived over those who traveled solo or in smaller networks. They also outcompeted those who stayed in one location, who were more likely to die out due to shocking weather or famine.[5] The hunter-gatherer style of living became ideal for survival. Its success in sustaining more people for longer allowed it to expand as a style of living. Networks were spread out wide and protected fellow kin while sharing their goods. To exist this way, these groups held values of reciprocation, generosity and collaboration.[6] They were spread into huge networks that worked together to meet their needs.

As the Earth warmed up with the rise of CO_2, domestication of land became more possible and we entered the age of the Holocene. Holocene is the geographical era that began after the last ice age, about 12,000 years ago.[8] Eurasia was land that was rich in easily reproducible indigenous plants, and animals that could be domesticated.[5] These conditions were perfect for farming. Some of the hunter-gatherers started settling down and became farming societies. This style of living could ensure survival better than the nomadic life and grew through assimilation of hunter-gatherers and outliving their nomadic peers. "Thus, early farming spread not because rational individuals prefer to farm, but because farming communities with particular institutions beat mobile hunter-gatherer populations in intergroup competition."[5]

Many of these shifts that happened from nomadic to stationary living influence our psychology today.

Geographical pressures are the first to help form the psychologies of any people. Rituals and social norms were (and still are) heavily reliant on the geography and landscape of the land. With ancient peoples that were mostly nomadic, that meant hunting, gathering and finding resources in new places, so they had to have a generalist view. They kind of had to know a little bit of a lot, to distinguish poisonous plants from non-poisonous ones, there had to be a general awareness of how to be in the relationship with the animals they encountered and for those they looked to for nourishment, how to kill, slaughter and cook them, and which spirits and gods could assure them easy passage, all of that would vary based on location. When I use the word "understand" here, I do not mean neocortical study or analysis, although there is no denying that played a part in the navigation of the times. I am including in "understand" a knowing that arises from sensing and feeling.

They had to sense and feel, therefore, understand, a little bit about the meaning of the moon, sun and stars and their relationships to what would be available to them, like what grew when or to help them travel. When settling became the better strategy, they narrowed in on what they needed to know. They only had to understand the cycles and spirits of the land they were occupying, what that land offered and what they would need to cultivate themselves. They only needed to know the animals in their area and the best ways to prepare these animals and how to domesticate them. In other words, their views got narrower.

Ceasing the nomadic life meant that rituals and attention shifted to connect to the particular land they inhabited and towards cohesion of the group. As these settled groups grew, they assimilated hunter-gatherers. This was a competitive function because these communities, with their domesticated animals and land full of vegetation, became easy targets. They were basically like an open buffet for the nomads. The strategies to survive became to invite their nomadic peers into the society mostly through new institutions like what we think of as marriage and launch defensive strategies to protect their property like what we think of as military. However, these defensive actions were not the only things that made them succeed in the inter-group competition; it was their rate of reproduction. Their settled lifestyle allowed and created the need for labor, encouraging sex for reproduction.[5] Here, we see "cisheterosexual sex itself becomes a means of productivity."[9] Through assimilating nomads through unions and increased reproduction rates, they literally outgrew hunter-gatherers, which led to their survival and eventually outnumbering nomadic peoples of Eurasia.

However, as these groups grew, new social norms were needed. These groups excelled because every smaller clan's survival depended on that of their neighboring clans. The combination of clans created kinship-based networks. Extensive cooperation became necessary.

Understanding the shift from nomadic to settled is important because of the psychological shifts that still exist today, like narrowing focus and increasing the need to expand or to scale up as a form of protecting territory (even if they did not consider land as something to be owned then). These shifts were appropriate and strategic, but are the seeds of the oppression we see today.

Scaling Up

In our culture today, growth, expansion, scaling up are seen as signs of success and are strived for. For our ancestors, it was a strategy for survival. Let's dive into how this strategy was further developed and implemented.

We are going to skip ahead many centuries. Those networks of small clans grew in population, and as they grew, there became more territory to protect. To maintain their size, they had to create norms, rituals, taboos and rites that "permitted larger communities, broader cooperation, greater production, and better command and control."[5] In other words, they had to create rules that would make the group more homogenous if they wanted cooperation in the scaling-up effort. One strategy in this project was what we would now see as natural hierarchies. Natural hierarchy was decided based on lineage. That makes sense to us now because it's been a long time understood as a norm, but that was a strategy, not natural human orientation.

Lineage-focused hierarchy ensured that the new chiefs were in relationship with all the clans. Someone could not campaign for the chiefdom; it was about who had the most connections to keep the group intact. In many large-scaled groups (that have been studied), the chief's primary function was to settle disputes between clans. Because they were interconnected to the clans in the network, they had the loyalty of the clans. The chief could be someone who had ancestral ties to major ancestral spirits amongst the network as well. So, let's say there is a network of four clans. There could be two cousins that are in line for the chiefdom, but one cousin is related to all four clans based on their father's lineage and the other only three. Because the one with all four connections meant they had more ancestors in common with more of the clan, they were better suited for the cohesion of the network and better suited for the chief. The chief's role was about restoring peace and harmony and to keep the network intact. Their energy went to interpersonal relationships and maintaining peace within networks. This is not to pretend or idolize antiquity as non-violent; it was plenty violent and varied.

Anthropologists note that ancient civilizations remained small due to disputes and ruptures between clans. Each time there was a split between clans, it made the whole group vulnerable.[5] To reduce conflict and increase loyalty, our cultural ancestors prioritized patrilineal lines so there was always a clarity on where loyalties belonged, so they assigned loyalty based on a person's father. So, if there was a dispute between two clans and someone's father and mother each came from one of the clans, they would align with their fathers. This shifts an importance to fathers, male lineage.

This process of scaling-up through patrilineal lines uplifts logic and strategy. Qualities such as nurturance, attentiveness, narrative keeping and sensing were feminized (becoming associated with the feminine), and are minimized to a lesser importance in the scaling-up endeavor. They still work to keep the cultural aspects of the clan, but not the structural. Basically, to scale up, you have to make some things more important than others. I don't know about you, but I feel the direct contemporary example of this in the non-profit sector, organizing world and the budding psychedelic-assisted psychotherapy industry. Sacrifices must be made for growth, and the sacrifices always seem to be the ones that are slower, more caring and relational. That is oppression enforcing that some needs, values, wants and interests are not as important as others in accomplishing goals and, therefore, can be dismissed.

Back to our ancestors. Scaling up also changed relations. Relationship to people, land and spirit.

The use of unions or marriages was a tool to maintain networks. Marriages between family members were usual and expected. This reduced the opportunity for rupture as they were ancestrally tied. Marriage was also used to create alliances and make peace between clans.[5] These unions are not about a family unit as we have come to see it now. Although I would argue marriage is still strategic.

Access to land was a reason people may marry. Land belonged to the society.[5] Whoever was in the clan belonged to the land and vice versa. This meant when clans merged with other clans, they did not lose their land, but instead had more access to land when marrying into or being overtaken by a neighboring group. With access to new lands also came access to the spirit of the land.

Most spiritual beliefs included land-specific gods, and ancestral spirits and spirits of the beings of the land. From neighboring clan to neighboring clan, their deities, rituals and rites were unique and intertwined with daily living. Spiritual ritual was intertwined with socializing and working. When new land was acquired and clans grew in network, unique spiritual beliefs did not interrupt that of the others. There was an understanding that their gods, ancestral deities and nature spirits belonged with the land and clan.

As clans intermarried, we see the mutation and creation of new deities and gods as they combine beliefs, traditions and rites. We also see that people may abandon their gods and deities and adopt those of their new network since they seem to be doing well for them. This was not seen as spirituality, religion or any special component of living, but central to group cohesion and belonging to land and each other. Rites and rituals that we now consider individual spiritual activities were part of the maintenance of societies.[5] As these societies of clan mergers scaled up, so did their gods. The more clan connections an ancestor linked together, the more important they became. The more important they became, the more powers they would have over smaller local ancestors. So local gods dealt with clan matters, while these bigger ancestors, deities and gods worked on behalf of the whole network. So let's bring back our cousins from earlier. The cousin with connections to all four clans may be connected through a great-great-grandfather. Because this great-great-grandfather connects more clans, he, over time, will be given more authority and power than ancestors who connect less clans.

Our current cultural understanding of spirituality and ritual is so far from these times it's hard to truly understand for myself. Especially rituals that induced orgiastic states. They were often engaged to expand consciousness.[10] Through movement like dance, singing, drumming and plant medicines (what we call psychedelics today), they could reach expanded states where their view widened and gifted perspective from land, cosmos, ancestors and spirits. But this was not deemed "spiritual use" or "healing use" as we have positioned them in the emergence of the psychedelic-assisted psychotherapy industry. "Shamans consulted the spirits of these plants for community guidance, for divination of hunting and weather patterns, to commune with ancestors and help make peace between warring factions, and, most elementally, simply to know and learn their ways."[6] These states were not exceptional; they were part of maintaining the cohesion, belonging and hygiene of the group; they brought solutions to group issues, not individual problems.[10] This is so different from our approach to spirit now, but the changes that come out of Christianity and cultural evolution help explain the gap.

We are about to go into a section about Christianity and its impact on contemporary psychology. As I live in this Judeo-Christian-dominated culture, I know the importance of understanding these concepts and their influence on how I perceive the world. Please take this in as an exploration of cultural evolution, not a discussion on the Judeo-Christian beliefs.

Christianity Out Competes

For the most part, most cultures looked similar to what's being described around the world. It is also the basis of Euro-asian cultural evolution, which was drastically changed by the introduction of Christianity. Muslim scholars described early Europeans as "white barbarians."[5] They were not that impressive. And yet, with time, as the early Christian's doctrine, force and wealth spread along Europe, these barbarians became a culture consumed with becoming orderly, disciplined and superior.

Monotheistic religions were a product of cultural evolution. As we just explored, to connect more people, their ancestors and spirits became more powerful. Gods that were once elements of nature are now human-like and powerful and exist outside of nature. They are also more powerful than local deities, spirits and ancestors. Christianity's foundation was that there was an omnipresent God that rules over all the universe and is deeply invested in the daily lives of humans, their thoughts and actions. This omnipresent God meant that they did not have to be connected to a particular land or group to have a connection to this God. This gradual shift from localized clan and land-specific deities comes with massive shifts in psychology.

For example, let's say my clan is within a network and we have our local gods who we communicate with and are engaged in ritual with throughout the day. And one day, we get into a dispute with another clan within our network which has their own set of gods. Our differing gods, taboos and norms may cause us to have different ways of how to settle the dispute, so we go to the chief who will invoke a shared god; we have to determine the right course of action to settle the dispute. Because this is a shared god, they out-power our local gods, taboos and norms. This settles our disagreement and reminds us of our loyalty to our shared god and, therefore, each other.

In what we now call Europe, we see this shift in the last of the Greco-Roman gods who became concerned with individual clans and their acts and doled out punishment for misactions. The last of the kinship-based Greco-Roman gods were already becoming more concerned with the moralities of individuals, which is not present in earlier deities of smaller societies. Their gods pivoted towards valuing the honor of a larger society, therefore, the individuals that make it up.[5] These larger gods became gods that could punish a whole clan if they ignored taboos. So, clans became oriented towards following the rules of the bigger gods rather than their local ones. Clan members began surveilling each other to minimize the chances of dishonoring the whole clan and spare punishment. This is an evolutionary shift from gods that were mostly called upon to bring good fortune, reverse bad fortune, or simply lit up the day or blew on a windy day. Henrich shares that historically, the chances of a group creating a chiefdom when they did not believe in moral punishment was zero, but when a society believed in punishment for moral wrongs, the chances of creating complex hierarchies grew by 40 percent every few centuries.[5] This is the fertile ground which grew Christianity. The fertile ground of big gods who punish.

These changes allowed for the rise of the version of Christianity that would later become the Catholic Church in Europe. There were many different types of these religions competing for the attention, hearts and souls of networks and clan power figures.

Around 200 BCE, we see these universalizing religions spring up with a focus on afterlives (what happens after you die), free will (that individuals can choose their own paths) and moral universalism (that there is a natural right and wrong).

These beliefs brought with them cultural incentives, and, till this day, societies that adhere to beliefs accompanied by a fear of punishment by a supernatural entity have less crime and increase productivity. Like, if the bigger god thinks killing is wrong, then individuals won't kill, even if they do not personally see an issue with killing. These new universal moral mandates decreased rupture between group members and allowed the group to get bigger in size. These are the cultural incentives needed for these societies to scale faster and wider than ever before.

These things may sound good since we live in a culture that strives for a moldable mass, but this is oppression. And the reason we have a hard time seeing it as oppression is because we see these things as natural and moral. But as we have just discovered, these morals are not innate; they are taught, they are conditioned, they are strategic. Universalism allows us to adopt oppressors' ideology as the right way to be and enforce it on others. That is oppressive. Using fear of punishment or punishing others who do not act how you want, is oppressive. This one will be controversial, but stay with me. Creating the concept of free will that makes you free from connection to place and people – disconnecting you from belonging is oppressive.

Breaking Up Clans, Building the Individual

So, the Christian church has a directive to scale up and, to do so, must create norms that could unify people of varying clans, beliefs and traditions. The "marriage and family program" of the early Christian Church, as Henrich affectionately calls it, was a strategy that created new structures and definitions for kinship.[5] This program had various initiatives. Henrich goes into full detail in the book; I will only highlight a few of their initiatives that are relevant to this exploration narrative. Please keep in mind that the psychological impacts of these structures were not planned; the structures were based on religious interpretation and a cultural evolution that was already primed for these shifts.

The first pillar I will discuss was creating a legitimate marriage. First, they elevated the importance of marriage over all other relations. They also did not recognize all unions, so some that may have existed prior were seen as invalid within the church. Some familiar ones that were no longer recognized were intra-familial marriages, such as cousins getting married. Because of the previous importance of lineage, many people around each other were somehow related. This meant that now it was expected that people had to travel far away to get married. The second pillar was that the church did not recognize multiple marriages. This meant not recognizing second marriages, and it meant monogamy was expected. This also meant less ties that connected differing clans to each other.

The other pillar we will cover was the shift in a legitimate family. Only the children from the legitimate marriage were recognized as being in a family.

Previously, children from other sexual partnerships were recognized as kin, and adoptions were very common. Even adoption of adults into a clan. These three pillars alone broke up large, intensive, kinship-based networks into smaller family units that were committed to this bigger god over kin and land, which made them loyal to a spiritual community.

With the new legitimate family structure, "the church released individuals from the responsibilities and obligations and benefits of their clans . . . creating more opportunities and greater incentives for people to devote themselves to the church and later to voluntary organizations."[5] In other words, maintaining connection was no longer the priority, being a faithful devotee was. This freed people to abandon kin and travel further away to find someone to marry and create a spiritually recognized family.

Prior to this, generations of clan members inherited land from previous generations; land was not owned. Selling land was "unthinkable because these territories are the home of the clan's ancestors, and deeply tied into the clan's rituals and identity."[5] And with the transfer of land, there was a transfer of authority. So, young people did not take charge of the workings of the clan until the elders died. So once an elder died along with maintenance of the land, the next generation was able to take up the roles they received to maintain the collective. Unlike contemporary culture where young people are expected to make a purpose or role in the world for themselves.

The church changed land inheritance with the Last Will and Testament, where a priest would sit by a dying person's bed and ask how they would like their possessions split up after their death. This was seen as basically their last chance to get into heaven. With the narrow scope the church had of legitimate family, people were restricted in who they could leave land and possessions to. This is how land became something you can own and privatize. The church became quite wealthy through the last will and testaments of patrons. People often left money and land to the church, with the idea that it was "redistributed to the poor" through the church's use. Sidenote: the church also made a fortune from all the pardons they gave to people who paid them so that they could continue being part of the church but did not want to adhere to all of these new rules.

With the assurance of their families' land stripped away, the need to find a spouse that is unrelated, and no longer having a role they knew they would inherit from elders, new Christians oriented themselves towards creating these for themselves through building personal wealth. This encouraged younger people to leave their clan with the support of their new faith. "How could they do this?" You may be asking. Well, because of the impersonal trust that came with Christianity.[5] Impersonal trust means that you can trust someone because of an association you share, rather than knowing them yourself. This meant that anywhere you went, as long as there were Christians there, you could trust them even if you did not know them or have familial ties to them. As opposed to clans that only did exchanges with those they were quite familiar with. Travel increased the pool for marriage, work and teachers to learn skills.

Without intensive kin-based institutions to organize production, provide security, and endow people with a sense of meaning and identity, individuals were both socially compelled and personally motivated to relocate, seek out like-minded others, form voluntary associations and engage with strangers.[5]

The nomads belonged to the earth, our clans belonged to their land, these new Christian individuals did not belong anywhere.

Feel Into It

Are you heartbroken yet? Feel into having the security of land and kin stripped away, making you into a lone wanderer.
What does this make you want to do?
How is this still happening now to you?
Check your hands, shoulders and jaw.

Practice to Intervention

I am heartbroken almost every session I have. Allowing myself to be heartbroken is a powerful ally in my work. In a culture that normalizes being stripped from belonging, our clients often do not recognize there is heartbreak to experience. I make sure to use this language when I feel it. Which is often. "That's heartbreaking." I notice with time, people begin to take their experiences more seriously as they keep having it reflected with such serious emotion.
What are the versions of being stripped from belonging that your clients experience?
Challenge yourself to notice when the feeling of heartbreak comes up in you when listening. Can you bring yourself to name it?

In the search to belong, these new individuals needed personalities to attract relationships that helped them feel belonging. "They become biased toward creating mutually beneficial connections based on their individual abilities, dispositions and characteristics."[5] In other words, making friends becomes important. This psychological shift is brought to you by impersonal trust, increased mobility, decreased connection to land and disassociation to clans. Practicing this new bias, Christians started their own clans now in the form of voluntary organizations. At first, these organizations were religious organizations. As markets became a way for individuals to create wealth, there was less and less connection between sellers and buyers. New voluntary organizations emerged, called guilds, changed this. Guilds are centered around skills and talents that individuals could take to market. Think of any contemporary accrediting boards or institution that essentially says you are trustworthy because they have given you the stamp of approval. These guilds included standards and codes to remain in membership and validated sellers in the marketplace. Individuals had to make themselves attractive to these guilds to receive invitations to become members and, once they were in, they must sustain membership by adhering to standards set by the guilds. In return, the guilds have to make themselves attractive, so people want to join. The guilds ensured certain rights and privileges were given to the individuals that fulfilled their obligations to the guild. This is the cultural introduction of individual rights.

Couldn't agree more with Rev. williams when she says the idea of rights "gives rise to the very policing that diminishes humanity by seeking to sort us into categories of relative entitlements."[11] The creation of rights only makes sense if a culture is focused on separating individuals that are deserving from those that are undeserving; rights are often property or privileges that can suddenly be taken away therefore is needing of protection.[5] Individual liberty created an implicit pact that an individual "had the right to be fed, but he must accept the physical and moral constraint of confinement."[12] The confinement here is of acting appropriate or desirable by the body that promises the rights. Thus, as Foucault writes, "liberty is an 'invention of the ruling classes' and not fundamental to man's nature or at the root of his attachment to being and truth."[12] Liberty is always conditional; it is based on the norms and expectations of the body that grants you liberty, and if they can give it to you, they will take it away.

This is a fundamental part of oppression, that your ability to make a life for yourself is based on those who have the power to validate you and, therefore, create the conditions you must adhere to. Today this may go without questioning because that is how our world works, but it's important to remember that this is an ideology that was created out of the necessity of displacement and lack of connection.

Feel Into It

What's it like to consider that human rights are made up? That nothing is actually owed to anyone? That nothing is owed to you? What happens to you? Can you stay with it? What happens in your belly? Express what comes up.

Practice to Intervention

I find myself in sessions where the pain someone is experiencing is actually about the betrayal that was felt by not having something they believed they deserved to have. Feeling as though we deserve something and did not get it in this culture is a major root of many of the reasons people come into therapy. Like, they are infuriated by a barista who did not make the right drink, or their boss who overlooked them or their parent who did not give them affection. Since I am clear, I am owed nothing and bring myself into the painful process of feeling that, I am less likely to get wrapped into the "injustice" of the experience and into the disappointment or rejection of it much quicker.

These guilds became the framework for other organizations. After the Protestant Reformation and the increased moral value of reading (recall Chapter 1), we see these guilds take an academic bend, springing up into universities. They became a location to philosophize, debate and learn theory. The structures that came out of these guilds were also replicated to create towns, cities, states and, much later on, countries and the bureaucracies created to control them. Populations became organized into groups created around their marketplace value. Schools that were initially only about reading the bible grew to incorporate military training techniques to teach skills that individual children needed to become attractive to voluntary organizations. This created an expansion in possible personalities an individual could have. "Traits got exaggerated or suppressed" based on what was marketable.[5] The marketplace later expanded to be more than a physical location to sell and buy goods; it included labor. Markets are an essential feature and are seen as the beginnings of the current World Economy, which gives rise to capitalism.[4]

I want to go on a small tangent with two notes. First, not everyone was welcomed to these voluntary organizations; they were exclusive. Secondly, because of the cultural evolutionary biases towards patrilineal lines and men, it was people socialized as men that were encouraged to make themselves attractive to voluntary organizations. People socialized as women were encouraged to make themselves attractive to men by learning and performing the socially desired behaviors of women. Success for these women was getting married. "In a culture that so dearly values the individual, love achieves the ultimate goal for individuals: to be united in mutual admiration, attraction or longing."[2] These unions were based on the personalities of the individuals. This is a big difference in the use of marriage, as we discussed earlier. Although this quote is speaking to a more current idea of love, it links to this root of making yourself marketable.

The combination of disconnected individuals searching for a way to make a living and voluntary organizations brought a lot of people to big cities where there were more opportunities. In 800 CE, there were 700,000 people living in cities with 10,000 people or more, while in 1800 CE, there were 16 million people living in cities of 10,000 or more![5] "Capitalism depends on something called growth," these cities exemplified that.[13] Capitalism's reliance on endless accumulation made it important that there was a constant stream of new technology, new ideas and then expansion of those ideas to new territories as a product for the market.

The West began to consider themselves more developed and evolved societies because of their large cities. The cities became a breeding ground of intellectuals and bureaucracies who philosophized about how to replicate their evolution in places they deemed "less developed." This sense of superiority spread throughout these European or European descendent nations (United States). At the same time, European cities were not the ones with the highest density of people, were not the only ones with written and spoken language across large swaths of populations or studied philosophy. Countries in Asia and in the Arab world had all of these.[4] However, they were not as militarily or technologically advanced according to European standards and, therefore, considered primitive or stuck, not modern.

This psychological shift moved progress to the realm of "possibility rather than a certainty."[4] In other words, if people do not labor to advance, they will become stuck or primitive like these other people. This is still a belief today that progress is the ultimate goal and will not happen if it is not made. But actually, things are always progressing, whether we do something or not. What we usually mean but are not saying is, "I have a belief about what progress looks like, and this is not it." This underlying unsaid part is what is oppressive. What we consider to be progressive is superior to that of another, and it gives us permission to impose our belief on them. But historical Europeans ignored that, in actuality, the civilizations they were calling primitive or stuck were existing at the exact time as they were. This smug and untrue belief was the foundation of the Enlightenment period.

Self-Titled Enlightenment Period Makes Competition Intellectual

What does it say when a historic period names itself? Self-absorbed. The Enlightenment period was just that. It was a period that solidified for itself that its new norms made Europeans and their descendants modern. The purpose of life shifts from being devout to being civilized. Civilized equals secular and modern. Enlightenment focused the mind on what can be seen, proven and replicated. In many ways, they decided what should be visible and what should be hidden.

In this time, we see scholars revisit formerly unexplored theories and philosophers. The propaganda of the time is that discovery becomes available to everyone, anyone could discover something or debunk what was previously believed to be true. Knowledge becomes competitive. This time solidifies the bias towards analytical minds and using them towards specific study or expertise. Narrow view.

Although there is a surface-level competitive feel, much of what was created during Enlightenment was a combination of thoughts. Multiple identical discoveries or inventions were made across the West at the same time.[5] In retrospect, it really showed the power of collective consciousness more than a boom of individual brilliance.

The illusion of intellectual competition combined with the longer days due to artificial light encouraged people in the cities of these "civilized" nations to work longer hours, going from 10–15 hours a week to 45–60 hours on average a week.[5] City infrastructure enabled this by incorporating clocks and light as adornment in public areas, but also to support a new culture that is oriented around using time wisely. The concept of working for wages becomes widely accepted, making time into money.[3] With wages, some characteristics become ideal, such as being patient, since you will not get paid right away, having discipline to produce work as expected and compliance to authorities, now including supervisors. This also orients every present moment towards a future reward.

Prior to these major cultural shifts, work, social and spiritual time were all interwoven. In older societies and still now in places not governed by Western ideals, "life was largely organized by natural rhythms- daily, seasonal, and annual- and 'the day' was organized by routine tasks. Moreover, there was often no distinction between 'work time' and 'social time,' since people socialized all day long while working."[5] Now, every moment could be used "wisely" as an investment towards an unknown future. Efficiency is becoming an ideal characteristic.

As a person who has deeply internalized and performs efficiency as a worthy characteristic, I am humbled by reading that the elders of the Dagara say that someone who is constantly in motion moving towards something is actually moving away from what they do not want to see or from what others do not want them to see.[14] The clock and time have become gods in themselves that keep looking towards the future in opposition to reflecting and understanding the past, for me and for our culture. As Malidoma Patrise Somé says, "The clock tells you everything and keeps you busy enough to forget that there could be another way of living your life."[14]

This oppressive time orientation is called chrononormativity. Chrononormativity is "the use of time to organize individual human bodies toward maximum productivity [by which] people are bound to one another, engrouped, made to feel coherently collective through particular orchestrations of time."[9] This concept pervades our ideas of what is normal, including things like eating meals. Europeans, in response to observing Indigenous people of the Americas grazing throughout the day, deemed that primitive and savage. To distinguish themselves as modern and civilized, they created mealtimes (breakfast, lunch, dinner). The concept of chrononormativity is also seen in psychology's obsession with developmental models that tell us when it is appropriate to have certain experiences. This is oppressive because it is another form of universalism that ignores there can be other ways to live, other needs to consider and then goes on to force it onto others.

The Enlightenment period campaigned itself and still is often misunderstood as a time of great knowledge sharing, but actually, the universities were private institutions that were not in the business of sharing but of hoarding secret information. This play between secret and public, center and other, grows out of this time.[15] It is here we begin seeing history retold not from the victor but fabricated from the self-appointed victor. Industries develop out of this othering. History, the study of their own nations, which included invented tales of glory, is one; others include economics, political science and sociology that studied themselves in the present. Later on there is anthropology, the study of people who were under colonial rule.[4] Within this period, the French Revolution shifts how we think of politics, including that people of a nation are citizens, not subjects. These studies help create norms in the West for their citizens concerned with remaining in membership, therefore appearing modern and civilized, which introduces a new type of surveillance.

With the invention of the lightbulb, public areas became illuminated. Now, at all times, people of the West were expected to adhere to "civilized and modern" standards. The surveillance that was once reserved to uphold honor and avoid punishment from big gods is now used to protect the aesthetic of being modern. So many desires or needs that may have been previously uninteresting were now seen as archaic, primitive and taboo. The task of surveillance was distributed from the bureaucracies to neighbors, teachers, employers and religions. The increased level of surveillance, including the isolation of individuals, through individual family units, brought a duality; playing the role of a good and honorable citizen in public while having secret lives behind the convenience of their single-family homes.[15]

Feel Into It

Let's feel into time.

Notice what happens in you when you read these questions. Right now, do you feel on time? Are you where you should be? Record the responses from your body and mind.

Practice to Intervention

The relationship between time and money is very clear in our profession. Whenever I have a session where I feel I was not too hot or did not do some amazing tricks, I tend to feel badly, like I wasted the person's time, and they may regret paying me. This may motivate me to work harder next time so that I feel that I have earned the money we agreed to.

What is your relationship to time? How do you see chrononormativity impact you? Your clients? Your work with clients?

Colonization as a Side Note

There will not be too much direct discussion of "big C" colonization in this book, but we have already done much exploration of the oppressive ideals that make colonization possible and how they are still perpetuated in subtle ways today.

However, we must touch on it a bit. European nations, while all of this cultural evolution is happening on their land, are terrorizing the lands and brutalizing the people of other territories, deeply impacting their cultural evolution. Combination of their beliefs that separate them from the rest of the world by claiming they are civilized and modern, that progress must be made, not experienced, and capitalism that means endless accumulation, they embark on the colonization of the planet. This colonization is actually an economic strategy connecting all lands, making territories into sellers, producers or buyers.[4]

Invasion is not new to human history. However, invasion of earlier cultures was focused on creating connections to reduce the chances of being overtaken. European invasion seeks actually to take over so they can subjugate and use who they have conquered while elevating themselves further away as superior and financially profiting. European (and their descendants) invasion is never about merging; it is always about extinction, extraction and increasing their own illusion of themselves. Can you name some current day examples of this?

Waging war is also a strategic tactic. England was at war for most of 1100–1900 CE.[5] War is useful in making people within a nation more obedient under the guise of cooperating and more likely to self-regulate and surveil each other.[5] War is the perfect tool to keep unity within a super scaled-up group by making an "other" to unite against.

Alice Sparkly Kat writes that famine is a strategy of colonizers "created with the intent of turning people into wanderers – of detaching people from the land to which they are attached."[15] And from this brief history I have singled out in this chapter, it is clear that this strategy to dominate the world is only possible because Europeans did it to themselves first. Haden, Middleton and Robinson generously remind us that

> when any group must be controlled and used, their gods, their religion, their land and their tools of survival must be taken away from them. These are all reflections of themselves and their inner being as well as a practical means to living. This must be done by force at first.[16]

Which is what happened to the ancestors of the colonizers.

In a video interview, Resmaa Menakem says that white people never dealt with their trauma and they are blowing it through the bodies of black and brown folks.[17] Without that honest review of their evolution, they believe they are using neocortical strategy, but they are actually limbically responding to a history they will not face. That refusal to look back limits the compassion needed for themselves or anyone else to believe that other worlds are possible. It actually creates numbness to their own suffering or the suffering of others. This subverts the view of life, making suffering an unavoidable fact of life rather than being able to see when it is created and preventable. This stance absolves them from any responsibility but also from healing from this traumatic past. We have theories of people of color about moving through generational trauma, including Post Traumatic Slave Syndrome by Dr. Joy Degruy. There is also Dr. Maria Yellow Horse Brave Heart, who studies, theorizes, writes and speaks on the historical trauma of indigenous people. People of Color know we have historical trauma, but our trauma is not what has bled out everywhere else. White people have quite a distance in this realm to go. Dr. Maria Yellow Horse Brave Heart says, "[O]ur purpose is to heal from the historical unresolved grief . . . historical unresolved grief is the grief that accompanies the trauma."[18] She is speaking to the specifics of indigenous people, but I think historical trauma and cultural evolution are very tied. And Europeans and their descendants have a lot of unresolved and unexplored historical grief, and we all suffer from this disconnect.

In their numbness, European colonizers and their descendants terrorized the planet, motorized by their belief in themselves as modern and superior and complete denial of their trauma. They have exported their historical trauma through violent control, and forced their cultural-specific psychology onto societies that were still kinship-based, still land-rooted and rich in the personal and collective spirituality and traditions that came with kin and land. This has completely destabilized cultures, erased tradition and unmoored people, making those places into "third world" or periphery nations and European nations into core nations in the World Economy. Core nation-states are the rule makers of how wealth happens; periphery are the laborers or the resources for core nations.[4]

In other words,

The Machine has made itself look beautiful by making other ways of life that have existed for tens of thousands of years look silly, shameful and uncivilized. But the truth is that the Machine must eliminate every alternative to itself and focus every attention on itself because it knows that its purpose is not to give life, but to suck the energy out of it.[14]

As these core nations scaled up, their power was directly tied to the financial wealth they possessed. To increase financial wealth, they stole resources. This form of economy needs an "other" to create the surplus of people at its disposal.[19] They steal people. They kill and sterilize bodies they find unuseful.

To help justify this mind-numbing abuse of people of color, and all peoples held hostage in systems of indentured labor, there had to be an extreme objectification, where people become less than human. They become "things," denied their own chosen relationships, spiritual feelings, cultures, rights, and even the right to their deepest souls as Christianity was imposed through intimidation and repeated acts of violence.[20]

While some people become primitive and stuck, some people become non-humans.

They also steal ideas. "The more ideas they absorbed, the more recombinations emerged and the faster innovation chugged along."[5] This innovation led us to the Industrial Revolution, where we cemented our hate for the planet as well as other people. "The view of industrializing capitalism sees nature as an adversary to be utilized and exploited."[20]

Final Note

I hope at this time you can see that oppression is not a one-time calculated event; it is a series of beliefs that build on top of each other over time. This took centuries of a cultural evolution made possible through the luck of land and the incorporation of many other traditions. When Europeans began telling their own victory story, their norms became inspirational rather than the strike of luck, violence and trauma it actually was. Through colonization, the shift of European psychology that was enforced on them and became their norms was rebranded as the blueprint for the modern human.

Many of the characteristics we value as normal in our current culture derive from this slow cultural evolution and are not natural human conditions. This evolution has brought us to the Anthropocene.[8] The Anthropocene is the geographical time we are currently in when humans are single-handedly creating our own mass extinction. We have increased the temperature of the planet, have assured the flooding of the land, and have an ongoing death wish for animals and plant life, all for the benefit of a few. While elites are looking to go to Mars to escape their mess, leaving everyone else to die, regular people are cheering them on. Betting on and arguing over which billionaire should settle on Mars first. This is why we must truly understand oppression because we work against our own interest with shallow comprehension. We cannot blame the elites alone for bringing about our extinction; it is also the internalized historical beliefs we utilize every day that encourages and sustains the Anthropocene.

We believe in the West, but also in psychotherapy, that all people just want to, or should want to work hard, do the right thing, trust institutions and systems, create new families, be a productive member of society, be an individual that sticks out from the rest, have private thoughts and secret desires, be cooperative and generous with strangers, find someone to love and the list goes on and on. But what I hope I have illustrated in this chapter is that these are not natural to being human; they are responsive to context.

The idea that there is a set of natural ways to be human reduces every person to being compared, analyzed and categorized, which we know is the function that happens in the neocortex. For this reason, I use neocortical supremacy as an umbrella that is expressed through white supremacy, capitalism, colonialism, racism, transphobia, cis-hetero supremacy, male supremacy, able-bodied supremacy, ageism and general human supremacy. Neocortical supremacy is oppressive because it squelches the space and possibility to accept beings as they are and allow for each being to live as they please.

Unlearning is the antidote I am proposing to neocortical supremacy. Unlearning is not about accumulating knowledge to be used to create something new; that's innovation and still neocortical. It is about using this amazing ability to be neocortical to critically investigate what we already believe, giving it context of how it came to be and observing our responses to it. Do we still want to practice this belief, or is it out of context and able to be retired in us? The practice of unlearning makes us flexible and detached from beliefs that are dead, that have outlived their usefulness, and open to what things are alive and in the present.

We've done some of the investigation of beliefs part in this chapter, and we will do some more in the next chapter, but observing if that belief is still alive or dead in you is something only you can do.

Practice to Intervention (For Black, Indigenous and Other People of Color)

This can be a ritual of honor. I know I do not honor the lives, entities and beings that were casualties to white innovation enough, so when I am reminded to, I like to take the chance. Here is a reminder for you.

Who and what would need to be in the ritual?
What would be performed?
Who would be named?
What role do you want the physical land you are on to play?
When will it take place?
These are not neocortical-strategic prompts. What tells you the answers?
The ritual may not happen soon, but the seed is sown.

Feel Into It

What is happening in you right now, considering this ritual? Record this.

Practice to Intervention (For European Descendants)

This can be a ritual of grief. I grieve how little grief happens in this culture. Take this moment to consider your ancestors and the numbness described above. Take a moment to recognize how it still shows up. Then take this as a grief nudge.

Who and what would need to be in the ritual?

What would be performed?

Who would be named?

What role do you want the physical land you are on to play?

When will it take place?

These are not neocortical-strategic prompts. What tells you the answers?

The ritual may not happen soon, but the seed is sown.

Feel Into It

What is happening in you right now, considering this ritual? Record this.

Citations

1. Lewis, T., Amini, F., & Lannon, R. (2001). *A general theory of love* (Reprint). Vintage.
2. Mesquita, B. (2022). *Between us: How cultures create emotions*. W. W. Norton & Company.
3. Guggenbühl-Craig, A. (1996). *Power in the helping professions* (12th ed.). Spring Publications, Inc.
4. Wallerstein, I. (2004). World-systems analysis. In *Duke University Press eBooks*. Duke University Press. https://doi.org/10.1215/9780822399018
5. Henrich, J. (2021). *WEIRDest people in the world: How the west became psychologically peculiar and particularly prosperous*. Picador Paper.
6. Maté, G., MD, & Maté, D. (2022). *The myth of normal: Trauma, illness, and healing in a toxic culture*. Avery.
7. Kolk, V. B. der, MD. (2015). *The body keeps the score: Brain, mind, and body in the healing of trauma* (Reprint). Penguin Publishing Group.
8. Haraway, D. J. (2016). *Staying with the trouble: Making Kin in the Chthulucene (experimental futures)* (Illustrated). Duke University Press Books.
9. Brown, S. (2022). *Refusing compulsory sexuality: A Black asexual lens on our sex-obsessed culture*. North Atlantic Books.
10. Fromm, E. (2006). *The art of loving* (Anniversary). Harper Perennial Modern Classics.
11. Williams, A. K., Owens, R., & Syedullah, J., PhD. (2016). *Radical dharma: Talking race, love, and liberation* (Illustrated). North Atlantic Books.
12. Foucault, M., & Rabinow, P. (1984). *The Foucault reader*. Pantheon.
13. Images, M. (2010). *Grace Lee Boggs and Immanuel Wallerstein in conversation – 2010* [Video]. Vimeo. https://vimeo.com/13407876
14. Somé, M. P. (1997). *Ritual: Power, healing and community (compass)* (1st ed.). Penguin Books.
15. Kat, S. A. (2021). *Postcolonial astrology: Reading the planets through capital, power, and labor*. North Atlantic Books.
16. Haden, P., Middleton, D., & Robinson, P. (1995). A historical and critical essay for Black women. In B. Guy-Sheftall (Ed.), *Words of fire: An anthology of African American feminist thought*. The New Press.

17. Jayson Gaddis. (2020, November 4). Resmaa Menakem on trauma & White body supremacy – Resmaa Menakem – 315. *YouTube*. www.youtube.com/watch?v=ouhKm_2bq5w

18. Woodland, E., & Page, C. (2023). *Healing justice lineages: Dreaming at the crossroads of liberation, collective care, and safety*. North Atlantic Books.

19. Lorde, A. (2007). Age, race, class and sex: Women redefining difference. In *Sister outsider*. The Crossing Press. (Original work published 1983)

20. Thanissara. (2015). *Time to stand up: An engaged Buddhist manifesto for our earth -- The Buddha's life and message through feminine eyes (sacred activism)* (1st ed.). North Atlantic Books.

Chapter 3

Scaled Up Societies

Things Start Changing, Fast

I hope you are a bit rattled. Anti-oppressive practice requires a willingness to be rattled. As Osho Zenju Earthlyn Manuel has said, "A society that does not examine itself is an unenlightened one."[1] In Chapter 3, we will continue to build off of the beliefs we have converted into facts about human nature and see how becoming nations and scaling up brought us Western Psychology. A culture of orderly, disciplined, innovative individuals who just want to be normal. We have already explored the historical context that erected our society. We saw that as these clans scaled up and became cities and then nations led by governments, the limbic longing for connection went from kin-based networks and transferred to these new conceptual associations.

Innovation is not a universal human trait; groups of people have often died from ongoing natural causes, which means we are not naturally innovators.[2] So, the evolution we are tracking is not consciously out of necessity. Henrich states, "[O]ur species' willingness to put faith in what we learn from others over our own direct experiences and intuitions" is a key ingredient in making sense of the shifts in how supernatural beliefs were able to move culture in such a drastic way in the West.[2]

In most pre-Christian societies, information was passed down from generation to generation. This information was interwoven between spiritual beliefs, rites, cultural taboos, norms, skills and labor, and there was not much incentive to change how things happened.[2] In kinship-based cultures, groups weren't motivated to innovate, but to sustain relationships, so norms changed slowly. Norms changed very quickly when networks were broken, and individuals with weaker relational ties had to stand out from the crowd to be invited into voluntary organizations.

DOI: 10.4324/9781003207054-4

Secularizing Christian Morality

The early Christian church could not ever have imagined how they would impact the world. Their "policies," Henrich writes,

> were gradually wrapped in rituals and disseminated wherever possible through a combination of persuasion, ostracism, supernatural threats and secular punishments. As these practices were slowly internalized by Christians and transmitted to later generations as commonsense social norms, people's lives and psychology were altered in crucial ways.[2]

Their campaign to convert everyone by force created individuals who dedicated their lives to "spreading the good news." Motivated by persuasion, ostracism, supernatural threats and later secular punishments, early Christians abandoned their kinship-based networks and went on to create their own lives. Empowered by their new mandates, protected by impersonal trust and looking to replace their loss of safety through kin, they moved to far away places in search of a partner and a career. Here, let's mark the new social norm of individuals searching to belong. This new expectation to be an individual searching resulted in a loss of ritual connected to land and rites focused on group cohesion and belonging. Here, let's mark a new social norm that spirituality is separate from daily life, land, work and societal belonging. To mimic that belonging, early classical-era Christians began creating voluntary organizations, such as churches and guilds. To remain in these organizations, to make themselves attractive to a partner, to create a career for themselves, they had to set themselves apart from the rest. Here, let's highlight the new social norm of needing to create an attractive personality. Skills that were formerly passed down for generations were now being learned through apprenticeships and market networks. With the increased competition between individuals to stand out, we see a new social norm of embracing and encouraging innovation and discovery. Here, let's note that being an innovator is a worthy personality. Innovation is the work of culture shifting. This is why culture changed so fast and continues to change so fast.

This adaptation is not genetic; it may have been spiritual, but it definitely was behavioral. This is an exploration of the behavioral adaptations individuals had to make to keep up with the quickly moving, innovative society and how these behavioral adaptations created long-lasting psychological changes.

The shifts may appear to be individual choice, but they were dictated by the church, then the guilds and later government. And all of this came from the belief of universalism. That there is an essential (see natural) right and wrong way to be. It begins with an omnipresent god who can see into your mind, read your heart, is very concerned with your actions and judges you at the end of your life. This means that everything you do now isn't about now; it is about later. Note this is a norm of the compulsion away from the present and towards the future. Seeing our every action as a credit towards control in some unknown future.

These right or wrong ways were first behavioral, via surveillance by community, but as the omnipresent god gained the ability to read minds and thoughts, self-surveillance arose; this is a psychological shift. This is the psychological beginning of having a private inner world, separate from an outer public performance. This inner world was, and could be, influenced by bad things. Maintaining spiritual inner wellness became the new task of the new Christian individual.

Remember, in the beginning, people were unable to read the doctrine themselves; they relied on the priest to guide them on what was right or wrong. Basically, they stopped sensing it for themselves. They essentially gave their lives over to the priests. Well, the elites did; everyone else heard the messages via trickle-down effect. The priest could tell you if you were on track for a good ending or not. If you weren't, they could coach you or confer with God on your behalf. This is a very Christian deity-specific characteristic: a deity "who was subject to persuasion by prayer, and who might intervene as supernatural force."[3]

Since not only actions could be sinful, but thoughts as well, going to authority to confess thoughts and desires became as common as confessing actual actions. Foucault describes this as desire turned into discourse.[4] When desire turns into discourse, your desires are no longer something felt in the body that propels you towards a satisfying action, but something to be investigated, analyzed, discussed and changed with the support of an authority figure; at that time, the priest. This resembles many therapeutic models.

The Protestant Reformation discouraged turning to the priest as interveners between God and individuals. The revolution was based on the belief that through reading, devotees could create their own connection to God. They could read for themselves how they should be. Therefore, no one could blame anyone else if they did not make it to the pearly gates. In a way, priests maintained some illusion that these individuals weren't totally alone. The reformation shattered that illusion. Individuals were totally responsible for their fate. Hard work became the pathway to heaven; it replaced confession as a purifier.

You could work hard to purify your thoughts and desires. You could work hard to make up for wrong actions. Stillness became the devil's playground. If there was a moment of stillness, you could study the Bible. All of your time should be occupied with being a good, God-fearing person. And the barometer of good was not in you; it was in the Bible. If you were not sure where you stood, work more, do something else, work harder. Work becomes a method of earning good character. It was expected that

all the poor who are capable of working must, upon work days, do what is necessary to avoid idleness, which is the mother of evils, as well as to accustom them to honest toil and also to earning some part of their sustenance.[4]

Hard work becomes an essential attribute to remain in society. These hardworking folks reduced crime in big cities, were more cooperative with others and produced a lot. Hardworking people, it turns out, are preferred to scale up societies.

Feel Into It

These are some of the Master's tools.[5] Audre Lorde writes about us being clear about how insidious oppression is because without that clarity, we end up intending to do something different but using the same oppressive tools available to us. Some of these tools seem fundamentally "good" because of society, but they are actually in alignment with oppression like:

- A search for belonging.
- Spirituality being separate from daily life.
- Personality needing to be attractive.
- Being an innovator is a desirable personality that deserves power and/ or leadership.
- Being future-oriented and forward-thinking.
- There is a right or wrong way to be.
- Desires should be thoroughly explored.
- Hard work brings purpose.

What comes up for you reading these? Sensations? Emotions? Which ones cause you to grapple? Share that with your group.

Scaling up shifted entire industries of philosophers from theorizing about the cosmos to imagining what it means to create the perfect cities and societies on Earth. They abandoned being in awe of the universe and unknown to studying how to control others. Prior to this one-size-fits-all all model of morality, morality was a choice elites made about whether or not "they want to have a beautiful existence."[4] However, it was not a choice regular people in these new Western cities could make; these universal morals became the expectation of everyone. Because we are geared towards staying in connection, and immorality is a risk to connection, we adhere.

Governing became a science and an art of control. It internalized the once religious and spiritual origins of a morality that was oriented around reaching for the perfect city in the afterlife for the task of bringing the perfect city on Earth.

Government value becomes clearly linked to how profitable the population is that they govern. The New World Economy becomes about making every territory into an actor in the market: sellers, buyers and producers. This turned nations into a competition wanting to become core nations that set the rules for the economy and profited the most from the rules they set, periphery nations that were resources for core states and semi-periphery that contributed the labor to core states in hopes they could become core states.[6] Finance and capital are future-oriented and it makes the future more real than the present. Finance becomes more real than actual life.[7] Governments take on the moral task of making heaven on Earth through perfect cities full of useful and profitable individuals. Because no matter what they say, states do not serve; they need servants.[8] Which is why people of a territory used to be called subjects. But in the new world economy, these territories become nations. They create some sort of history of what has happened within fictitious boundaries that have not always existed. They fabricate some set of characteristics that are unique to the nation but expected across the nation.[6] And reiterate some higher purpose for their becoming.

In other words, Capitalism, as Noah Harari writes and Gabor Maté quotes, "now encompasses an ethic – a set of teachings about how people should behave, educate their children, and even think. Its principal tenet is that economic growth is the supreme good, or at least a proxy for the supreme good, because justice, freedom, and even happiness all depend on economic growth."[9]

To solidify this, the judicial systems of these emerging Western cities convert moral codes into judicial law. These beliefs, once based on religious ideology, become secular. They become social norms disassociated from their religious origins and embraced as the rights of citizenship and signs of civility and modernism. The dissociation increases over time as the modern human is also a non-religious human.

Protecting the Perfect City

What was once surveilling becomes policing. Nation-states are "the only legitimate users of violence and should possess the monopoly of its use. The police and military are the prime vehicle of this monopoly."[6] Policing comes with authority and borrowed power to remove someone from civilization. Police became the eyes and ears of the government to find and punish those who are not proving themselves profitable to the perfect society. Police are also the laborers that work to maintain the aesthetic of the perfect city, removing those not performing the right way into confinement. This was also purposeful in deterring uprisings and disappearing people who opposed the oppression they received. Can't help but recall kin-based network chiefs, whose job it was to make peace amongst groups and how different this orientation is to that.

What to do with the differently abled, aged, mad, resistant? Confine them and make them useful. "Forced labor and the prison factory appear with the development of the mercantile economy."[4] As markets expand, the need for laborers expands as well. Hospitals and prisons become the punitive leg of the judicial system based on religious, moral codes that assure laborers for the markets. The staff of these facilities create the profession of the doctor. They use two main strategies to fix the morally corrupt people that have been captured: they either put them to hard work, expecting the hard work to purify them, or they isolate them.[4] The strategy with isolation was to completely ignore them until they were ready to behave in desired ways. The underlying belief is that individuals should control or dispose of their desires and impulses for the expectations of authority, and if you cannot, you are not seen as a human worth attention or care or even the bare minimum of deserving acknowledgment. Through these strategies, captives are trained on how to do emotions.

The hospital becomes a moral institution responsible for punishing and correcting moral delinquents. Individuals were released once they have proven their recommitment to work or to doing what is expected of them. These people being "evil fakers" was embedded in the word lazy, first seen in English in 1540. It originally meant "someone who disliked work or effort."[10] These "punitive mechanisms serve to provide an additional labor force"[4] by correcting their moral flaws and making them useful again. Sometimes, that meant returning to become a "productive member of society," but also, the work they were forced to do while held captive was often literally profitable in the marketplace for the institutions. As in making in and selling goods from these institutions. Slave labor through imprisonment is not new or a 13th amendment introduction; it was embedded into the system from the beginning.

While in custody, these individuals also become the first data study participants. Research on "human behavior" begins in these coercive and cruel institutions. Human behaviorists begin to create "the delinquent," the person whose whole life leads them to idleness.[4] Data collection to classify people or make them into cases for predictive calculations begins in these institutions. This practice is soon broadened out into society at large. Society becomes a mass of data.

Feel Into It

Notice the thoughts, sensations in the body, feelings that happen in response to this question:
Do you work hard enough?
Express them.

Practice to Intervention

Think about how regularly we hear, "they are choosing not to do the work." Our industry has not strayed much from our origins.

In the next few weeks, notice when you feel a client is not "doing their work." How did you feel before making that proclamation to yourself or to others out loud? What happens after?

I know this happens when I feel I am working so hard to "fix" someone and they aren't showing signs of change in the direction I expect. I get frustrated and begin feeling resentment that I am "wasting my time" (recall Chapter 2). I will often find myself sitting very forward and my hands are gripping something, either themselves, another part of my body or the seat. Once I make the proclamation and make it about their lack of effort, not my disappointment in the lack of gain I have made, I feel off the hook. And sometimes more than off the hook – that they deserve their suffering. That is hard to write and share, but it is important to say the "bad" things too.

Escaping Death: Norms, Health and Discipline

As psychotherapists, it is so important we explore our culture's moral value given to people who are disciplined, people who are healthy and people who are normal. Because quite often, the people who come in to see us don't think they are any of those things (even when they actually fit the bill). And honestly, they never will be any of those things, but neither will we, because these ideals are made up. We must shatter our own attachments to these ideals so we do not collude with our society when our client comes in asking us to help them have discipline. According to Foucault, discipline came about as a way to control the masses. He calls the science of controlling the masses bio-power.[4] Therapy is definitely in the science of bio-power. In bio-power, life itself becomes something that can be calculated. This makes the tasks of hospitals, prisons and other agents functioning on behalf of the government to create a "docile body that may be subjected, used, transformed and improved."[4] This was possible because, for the first time in human history, trying to control death became the objective of power. Death was no longer something that was random; it could be controlled.[4] Death was always something that could be induced by people in power, but what was new for the first time was the idea of postponing death, delaying death. And this new science made it so that death was controlled so they could bet against it for financial projections and political agendas.

However, this data is speculative as Kat writes. It has no real value; it is a creation of averages, comparison of behaviors and is all to move towards the goal of production.[7] This new field created experts in the human condition. Using the data they collect, their evaluations of and comparisons to other bodies, this new field calculates how to manage life.[4] This means life is not wild, unimaginable and full of surprise. It pulls norms out of their contexts of being an organic response to needs, environments, spirit and history but something that can be dictated via calculations and, therefore, can be measured.

Remember, previously, norms grew out of cultural necessities; these new norms, created out of this new industry, were created to increase the utility of all individuals in the society. It is a powerful tool not because it forces people to obey after they have strayed; that is what the police, the hospitals and prisons are for. These new norms are for the general population that will never interact with these institutions. It is powerful because it spreads "ideas about what is good."[4] Good keeps you belonging to the perfect city, to modernity and to civility. This is an evolution of the Protestant Reformation directive to be "good" people.

These new norms and the analytics that support them are used to calculate how to increase the number of useful members of a society and increase the longevity of their lives. The new task of good society members is not only to work hard but to stay healthy. It's weird to think of being healthy as oppressive. Being healthy is built on ideals that do not come from a place of connection but come from directives to stay useful. We hear it still today with ageism or hate for the disabled body. People casually say the worst thing they could ever be is "useless;" that is because our lives have no value if they cannot serve the state in the West.

Prior to the 17th century, a person who possessed an "erect head, taut stomach, broad shoulders, long arms, strong fingers, a small belly, thick thighs, slender legs and dry feet"[4] (yea, dry feet) was the mark of a perfect soldier and would be recruited into service. Later on, our mad scientist doctors realized that they could make anyone into the perfect soldier. So they trained and studied how to force bodies into soldier bodies. Through the success of this model, the perfect soldier became the model for the perfect body. Bodies became machines; this was later solidified during the Industrial Revolution.

The other influence on creating the perfect body was the othering of other bodies, like African bodies, who were categorized as uncivilized beasts[11] and used as the measure of the worst possible body. The creation of the perfect body is an act of violence ideologically that is then reinforced systemically and interpersonally.[11] This creation of the perfect body at the expense of other bodies solidifies the cultural evolution towards white supremacy by naming white bodies as normal bodies; it also named thin bodies, abled bodies and gendered bodies as normal.[11] This is used to justify their violation of other people.

Health, in name and in action, has always existed to abuse, to dominate, and to subjugate. The medical industry, the health care industry, and the diet industry all exist to maintain a culture intended to "discipline" those whose bodies refuse to – and, for many, simply cannot – conform to the standards of health.[11]

These norms under the guise of health were mistaken as a demonstration of the government's care for their citizens. What they actually were working on was increasing life expectancy so people could work longer. Life expectancy was tackled in three parts: increase the length of life with a new emphasis on hygiene and health (discipline) because having good health was simply a matter of discipline. The second part was an increased attention to sex as a mechanism of reproduction (self-regulation), showing restraint. And the final part was assuring more children made it to adulthood (control), exercising more control over children. The government cannot be everywhere, so these three goals are exported to the family units and medical clinics. The expert doctors that once were restricted to big city hospitals go on to open small practices in towns all over the West, taking the new norms with them.

The family unit is the primary actor of the government's will to ensure that children grow to become "functional members of society." And these families were being surveilled by neighbors, doctors and schools. The family is primarily the one responsible for "transmitting the requirements of society to the growing child."[9] The second transmission comes from schools. Schools that were once designed to ensure morality through learning to read the Bible, transform to do more. Schools borrow techniques from the military, from the prisons and hospitals that utilize humiliation, fear and punishment to make disciplined children.[4] Parenting became a hot topic; literature after literature advised parents that their children were just blobs of nothingness that needed to be beaten into shape. That shape should be decent people who possessed discipline, displayed self-regulation and were easily controlled. And later, during the Industrial Revolution, the schools changed again to include preparing these children to become laborers.[10]

How and why did all of these people go along with all these new rigid and cruel ideas of how to be? You got it; they were already headed this way due to fear of punishment or fear of being reported on via surveillance or fear of being confined in a hospital or prison, or fear of being shunned or kicked out of a voluntary organization, including jobs and, of course, fear of eternal damnation. Lots of things to fear.

Fear of punishment being a driver to participate is a uniquely Western concept. Henrich describes the findings of a series of studies where they explored cooperation fueled by punishment. Globally, participants who were punished for their lack of contribution to an activity went on to seek revenge, making them less likely to cooperate with strangers. For W.E.I.R.D. people, the more punishment they received, the more they wanted to cooperate with unknown participants.[2] Those fears that drive us to go along with this cruel new world do not need to be named or directly discussed to motivate cooperation; through cultural evolution, it is the quiet engine that runs unnoticed.

Fascination with how to create a sense of constant surveillance to avoid punishment was the basis of a whole industry of architecture. The panopticon, a focal image of Foucault's analysis of the time, was a model that arrived out of this new industry.[4] Architecture that once was mostly for aesthetics, making things beautiful, was now utilized to make cities more productive by increasing surveillance. The model was originally designed for a prison; however, it was absorbed into other types of city planning and development models.

Panopticon would look like this: a huge tower in the center of a plot of land. The tower is surrounded by buildings with rooms/cells housing people held captive. Each of the rooms/cells have two windows, one facing the center tower and one on the opposite side of the cell for light. A guard could sit in the tower and be able to see into all the cells. But the reason the model was studied was not the accessibility to view into the cells; it was that even if there was no guard in the tower, they expected the people held captive in the cells would self-regulate because they could never be sure when there was a guard looking in or not. This is ultimately an architectural recreation of an omnipresent god.

This never-ending possibility of punishment makes Westerners preoccupied with appearing disciplined. For context, discipline was once an oath designated for monks, for people who chose to dedicate their lives to renunciation and a religious life, not to become more useful. Discipline, like morality, was a personal decision in earlier times. Discipline was a strategy that a person implored towards what they personally found beautiful and divine. This was an intrinsic idea, of course still influenced by the cultural norms that informed individual pleasure and prioritized aesthetic beauty. Sadly, the discipline being discussed here is not that; it is generated and enforced externally towards health and norms that are constructed to make individuals profitable to the government, not about living their best life. This discipline is not about a person choosing and committing to the beauty they want to experience in their life, it is about forcing people to conform to a certain set of ideals not decided by them. And in the West, if you try to choose not to care for your life in a way acceptable to the state, you will be detained and exiled from society.

Feel Into It

Are you healthy? What makes you feel healthy right now? How do you feel unhealthy right now? List it out.

Are you disciplined? What makes you feel disciplined right now? How do you feel disciplined right now? List it out.

What comes up for you being asked to respond to these questions? Record those, too.

Go through your list. How many of them are feelings in your body that you are experiencing right now?

Practice to Intervention

So many of my sessions are, in some form or another, about someone feeling not disciplined enough. However, the more I am aware of my internalized drive to be healthier, be more disciplined and recognize it as a cultural issue, I have space to recognize that nothing is wrong with me. The more I accept that nothing is wrong with me, the less I collude with clients that something is wrong with them. I become more curious about the cultural beliefs and narratives that are in the space between us, and I name it. I also become curious instead about how their strategy is a good one, not an unhealthy one. Like with RL. At the beginning of our work, I agreed that they needed more discipline to stop doing drugs because that was unhealthy. I had no other frame other than that one to see it in. When I shifted away from believing there was a right way to be, I stopped colluding with them. Instead, I became curious. The collusion blocks curiosity. My curiosity made space for curiosity in themselves, and I can only hope that in time, that we did not have, it would have brought some compassion towards themselves. And that would have been satisfying work.

Building the Western Psyche

Here, we have landed at a crucial creation of current Western psychology. After being extracted from kinship-based networks individuals have to compete to build a life from scratch; the need to make oneself attractive to voluntary organizations becomes a major motivator of life. Those organizations evolve to governments that one must work to remain in membership; if not, one will be exiled to confinement. This work not only includes being a productive member of the society but proving a commitment to the longevity of your ability to produce by avoiding death and presenting oneself as disciplined and healthy. Since health and discipline are externally judged, a performance of these attributes becomes linked to belonging. And belonging is survival for this species.

"The presentation of a social face or mask relies on the existence of a hidden backstage in which actors can relax and prepare, negotiate and critique their roles."[7] This development of a private life with internal turmoil becomes the psychology of the West. Creating a backstage. This new expectation to perform fragments us. The front of the stage is our performance for the world. And in this society, we want the performance to remain consistent; we want people to be predictable, not complicated and nuanced. But the more consistently we must perform, the more gets pushed backstage.

If someone were to ask, "Why isn't that person saying anything?" In the West, they are more likely to hear in response, "They are shy," which says something about how that person *always* is, as opposed to more collective cultures where they may say instead, "No one asked them anything," which is about how they are responding to the situation. "In many cultures, people consider their emotions to be 'negotiated' with the social environment, rather than leading a separate life inside them."[12] Backstage can also be called the shadow, which is "where unacceptable parts of ourselves dwell, the places that we can't, or don't want to, see and feel, and so we therefore deny."[13]

So, you mean to tell me having an inner world is a Western concept and not a human trait? Yup! Our society made it necessary to create an inner world. If you are wondering what this means for our whole field, stay tuned.

The variety of personality in Western society is due to the ongoing development of new roles one can play in the society. People cultivate certain characteristics and diminish others based on the niche they want to belong to. In smaller, uncolonized, non-capitalistic societies, people are generalists and do not need to prove they have a personality matching the role they "plan" to play in society.[2] In other cultures, it is also expected that kin act differently depending on the context. These contexts range from the difference between speaking to an elder and a peer to the season and the rituals and rites associated with the season.[2] This is very limbic: being in a dance with the environment, being impacted and shifting based on conditions. However, in the West, "these cultural evolutionary pressures have fostered a rising degree of dispositionalism."[2] Because "analytical thinkers hate contradictions," dispositionalism is the orientation that people are consistent no matter the context, that people should always be "themselves."[2] And themselves can only be one thing.

There are two expressions of dispositionalism. The first is cognitive dissonance. Cognitive dissonance is the inability to tolerate our own inconsistencies, which makes us avoid looking at information that is incongruent with how we want to present ourselves and our society.[2] The second expression of dispositionalism is Fundamental Attribution Error, which is that we can make guesses about the internal landscape of a person based on their behavior regardless of context.[2] In other words, we do not look at the environmental, social, historical or relational surroundings of individual behavior; we see individual behavior as a direct reflection of their internal world.

When we say "ignorance is bliss" here, we mean it! Ignoring incongruencies in ourselves and others allows us to maintain the appropriate performances demanded by culture. The creation of a secret, private place that stores untouchable thoughts, emotions and desires allows us to maintain the appropriate performances also. But, of course, our culture has a solution to the problem it created. Confession.

Although the Protestants gave us an out, confession returns in the form of therapy! Not that Catholic priests went anywhere; they actually increased their accessibility to the general public – recall early priests only spoke to the powerful and wealthy. Confessing returns as a way to purify oneself of the inconsistencies.

"The liberal hero is always an honest hero, even – or especially – when he does reprehensible things."[7] Absolution can now come from honesty, no matter the action that is done, even ones not done but thought. What was secularized here is that along with God, Satan has access to our thoughts as well, and if we are having desires that conflict with norms, instead of it being about unrealistic and oppressive norms, it is about the individual and what lurks in them. It might be an evil invasion or, worse yet, we are unhealthy, deep inside. The belief that we cannot trust ourselves, that we need to look outside of ourselves for support in deciphering our inner happenings, is basically the field of psychology. It also is much of raising children in this society. This may be a familiar scene: a child is tantruming in the supermarket, and a parent tells their child, "Oh, you are just hungry," which is not a neutral observation but actually training the child towards an inner state that the child is not yet aware of. They are saying, "I know you think you are upset, but deep inside, you are really hungry, so your performance is inappropriate, and I am the authority, so I know more about your insides than you." This is one tiny example of how we teach children to disconnect from their body and learn the "right way" to be; we will discuss this more in Chapter 4. But this disconnect does not end in childhood.

This disconnect drives many people to therapy. To find out why their feelings do not match how they think they should feel or to understand what is wrong with them, that they cannot be disciplined or that they cannot keep up with their work or to find their authentic self or to find their purpose in life or to find love or to stand up to their boss. And this industry welcomes them with open arms, confirming that *there is* something wrong and promising we will help them figure it out. All of this performance, secret lives, cognitive dissonance and fundamental attribution error inform much of the field of psychology. It is not because we are cruel (well, not purposefully, and well, not most of us), it is because we believe them to be human nature. That people are naturally these ways; again, that is not true. We have been conditioned these ways, some of us longer than others.

We see cultural cognitive dissonance at play when so much of what is seen as taboo within the West is acceptable when in power. It is taboo to be an angry child, but it is expected to be an angry boss. It is taboo to rape people, but it is ok if you are a soldier overseas or drunk. It is taboo to have sex with a child or someone related to you, yet the rate of child sexual abuse climbs. Wanting to be polite, not wanting to talk about touchy subjects and turning towards more pleasant things are a few of the many ways we sustain our collective cognitive dissonance. However, we live in a traumatized and traumatic society; if we were to tune in to all of it, our analytical minds would just burst (I know mine has). So undoing cognitive dissonance is not about seeking trauma porn through Western news outlets; it's being open to the truth, all of it that you are present to. That when it presents itself to you, you do not turn away or hide.

Feel Into It

Big breaths. That was a lot. What is staying with you? How is it showing up?

Do a body scan. Notice where there is holding/tension/tightness. Where is there flow, easefulness, relaxation?

Do you know something about these sensations in these places? Share your observations.

Citations

1. Manuel, Z. E. (2015). *The way of tenderness: Awakening through race, sexuality, and gender.* Wisdom Publications.
2. Henrich, J. (2021). *WEIRDest people in the world: How the west became psychologically peculiar and particularly prosperous.* Picador Paper.
3. Ware, J. (2023). Searching for an abolitionist spirituality. In A. Crawley & R. Sirvent (Eds.), *Spirituality and abolition.* Common Notions.
4. Foucault, M., & Rabinow, P. (1984). *The Foucault reader.* Pantheon.
5. Lorde, A. (2007). The master's tools will never dismantle the master's house. In *Sister outsider.* Ten Speed Press.
6. Wallerstein, I. (2004). World-systems analysis. In *Duke University Press eBooks.* Duke University Press. https://doi.org/10.1215/9780822399018
7. Kat, S. A. (2021). *Postcolonial astrology: Reading the planets through capital, power, and labor.* North Atlantic Books.
8. Somé, M. P. (1997). *Ritual: Power, healing and community (compass)* (1st ed.). Penguin Books.
9. Maté, G., MD, & Maté, D. (2022). *The myth of normal: Trauma, illness, and healing in a toxic culture.* Avery.
10. Price, D., PhD. (2022). *Laziness does not exist.* Atria.
11. Harrison, D. L., & Laymon, K. (2021). *Belly of the beast: The politics of anti-fatness as anti-blackness.* North Atlantic Books.
12. Mesquita, B. (2022). *Between us: How cultures create emotions.* W. W. Norton & Company.
13. Thanissara. (2015). *Time to stand up: An engaged Buddhist manifesto for our earth -- The Buddha's life and message through feminine eyes (sacred activism)* (1st ed.). North Atlantic Books.

Part 2

Reconnecting to and Engaging the Limbic

Chapter 4

Familial Execution

Welcome to Chapter 4. So when we last left off, we had this society full of humans who have a public performance and a private shadow. "In each culture, caregivers teach their children the emotions that support the cultural norms and values. Having these emotions makes you part of your culture."[1] This chapter, we will explore how the emotions we perform for public go in the public pile and what goes in the private one and how the family unit is responsible to teach us which is which. We have seen how the individual was created; now we get to see how this concept of individuality is maintained.

On Being Animals

As I've mentioned before, we are in the age of the Anthropocene, and that means we tend to focus heavily on human-to-human interaction. The Anthropocene is the unofficial current epoch. This epoch is split from the Holocene (see Chapter 2) because humans (anthro) have become the driver of the sixth mass extinction expected to occur on planet Earth, as far as scientists can tell. In other words, humans have begun actively causing our own extinction through our self-centeredness. It is dated as beginning in the 1950s. It is estimated by 2100, there will be more than 11 billion people on the planet; this includes a 9 billion people increase between 1950 and 2100, 150 years of rapid growth and extended lifespans.[2] It is common to hear people blame technology for this disaster. We attribute the current and ongoing climate disaster that accompanied this epoch to machinery. I'd argue, we have simply created technology that rose to the task of the cultural evolutionary path the West has been on for the last 2,000 years. "The relocation of peoples, plants, and animals; the leveling of vast forests; and the violent mining of metals preceded the steam engine."[2] So our technology is making it quicker and more effective, not differently motivated. Although this is a global experience, based on all I have shared so far, I hope you understand when I focus in and say that this race towards extinction is the result of the self-centeredness of Western society and those that have adopted the practices and values of the West. This human centricity keeps us narrowly focused and we

DOI: 10.4324/9781003207054-6

ignore our species as mammals or as animals at all. Animals that are sharing the planet, not ruling it. Let's dive into the animal we named human.

Feel Into It

Different identities will have completely different intellectual, historical and embodied memories of this word usage in the question I pose below. These memories will impact how much or little they can feel this prompt. Let that be part of what can come up in your group discussion and hold that this is a moment to feel into it in your body and not to theorize it.

What happens in you when you are reminded that we are animals? Notice how your body responds to being called an animal.

What do you think distinguishes humans from other animals or nature? Has any of that been impacted by the last three chapters?

Brains evolved with time and with species. The reptilian brain, the oldest brain according to what we know now, allows us to do the fundamental functions of living, like breathing, eating, excreting and responding to life-threatening incidents. This brain primarily is focused on survival. It is usually associated with fight, flight and freeze, but it's actually the power center. It sorts out tiny, seemingly insignificant but vital procedures like regulating the chemistry of our blood. That is a very complex and sensitive calculation, and unless something goes wrong, we do not even acknowledge it is happening. As mammals came into existence, another part of the brain developed, the limbic brain. This brain brought on new abilities that allowed more interaction with the environment. With it came skills like caring for young, pleasure, play as well as vocal communication, not necessarily like dialogue, but the ability to communicate states.[3] The newest part of the brain, the neocortex, is seen in more recent mammals. This brain is where reasoning, planning and communication through symbolism happen. This is where the idea of will and choice exists. Our overreliance on this part of the brain is what mostly differentiates us from our other mammalian family. In other words, most other animals cannot choose if they want to follow their instincts. They have an instinct, they follow it. Gabor Maté says this beautifully, "No other species has ever had the ability to be untrue to itself, to forsake its own needs, never mind to convince itself that such is the way things ought to be."[4] And like our mammalian family, the need we need most, is to stay connected.

Like them, we thrive in packs. Not only do we need others to thrive, but our physical systems are geared towards connection with the world around us. Mammals are organized towards protecting relationships, especially the ones we are most genetically related to. The human drive for connection is less of a choice; it's biological. To understand this, we need to explore the limbic "brain" or system. This part of the brain, which is sandwiched between the "reptilian brain" and the neocortical brain, is a powerhouse in its own right.

Indus River Dolphins who echolocate have a lot to teach humans about the ways we are connecting without conscious effort, which is the domain of the limbic brain. When they echolocate, make sounds/vibrations, they are using it to locate themselves in the world.[5] Sure, we can focus on them finding food, but it is also about feeling connected; it tells them where they are. These vibrations bounce off of surrounding beings, return to them and now they know who and where they are. Indus River Dolphins may find themselves in unfamiliar waters, but they themselves are never lost. That is the power of the limbic brain. The human limbic system senses around us and collects information about where we are and how to be. Humans are doing this at all times, with or without awareness.

Losing the Pack

When early Western societies were made up of large clans (still happening in other parts of the world today) the limbic system had a lot of data to tell an individual about who they were and where they belonged. We all "functioned within a broad circle of attachments, the multigenerational clan, where consistent affection was modeled, encouraged, and shared."[4] People had sex, and people with uterus' gave birth and then a collective care of the birthing parent and child began. The other biological parent was insignificant and would drift off.[6] For so long, matrilineal connection was all a child could rely on because patrilineal lineage was unnecessary. We know that who we now would generalize as women (either due to their "anatomy" or the roles they occupied) would care, tend to, raise, teach and protect all their children and that of those in the network. Children's care was a collective responsibility, much like all other clan-sustaining activity, like farming, hunting, meal preparation, ritual leading, etc. In that system, when young people echolocate using their limbic systems, they had multiple ways of identifying themselves. Through their relationship to their many caregivers, many peers, their elders, their ancestors, spirits, deities and their land, young people knew who they were and who they would become. Again, I am not looking to romanticize and ignore what were pretty brutal times, as well.

Feel Into It

I just love that visual of a child echolocating. A deep longing rises in me with a warmth in my chest and cheeks and a smile on my face. It makes me want to reach out whenever I think about it. How about you? What happens in you? Do you know this longing? Can you let it just be?

Practice to Intervention

I've heard this said a few times in different settings and different ways: "note what people come to you for." Generally, it is used to motivate people to recognize a skill they possess that is valuable to the marketplace. But with echolocation, that shifts in meaning for me. I imagine in a collective society, what people come to you for teaches everyone around you the role you will play in the community. It says something about you, and the community reflects that back and honors it as who you are, not what services you can provide. I can definitely see a connection between someone ringing out who they are and nothing bouncing back to them that signals recognition and it creates a sense of being lost. If I think of ringing out as intuition, something that does not go through the thought process and the bounce back being an affirmation of that intuition, then the community's recognition is not only saying, "Yes, we see you," it is also saying, "What you know about you is right, trust that." This continuous loop in my imagination would make it hard to feel lost.

When I consider client issues through this lens, my empathy grows and so does my heartbreak. Are there clients you work with in which this shift or perspective would change how you see them and their "issues"? Write them down – reread these notes before your next session.

As clans began scaling up, a movement towards patrilineal superiority arose, a logical and strategic norm that narrowed who children were oriented towards. This is an example of aligning ourselves with the neocortical brain, leading to a culture that "promotes analysis over intuition."[3] This created an imbalance of new and gendered behaviors and expectations. Reducing the role of the limbic brain to "feminine attributes" like nurture and tenderness while elevating "masculine attributes" such as logic and aggression.[7] Lineage was now traced through patrilineal lines to reduce infighting and create a sense of logical loyalty between people within a lineage.[8] To increase collaboration, marriages were arranged, making potentially child-bearing bodies an object to own as it would increase the size of the clan and could unite clans within a network or new additions to a network. Although the unions were happening, they didn't mean instant family. When their wedded were away, the feminized group members were still collectively raising their children and the other children of their wedded as well as the children of their kin. Raising children was not a job as we see it now, it was what happens when young people are around, no matter how they came to be around.

Increases in clan and network size was initially to protect this way of life, intended to reduce infighting by assimilating clans in. With growing populations, the early Christian church isolated family units in the hopes it would create more control, order and civility. Think about it, trying to control a group of 1,000 people is easier when you control every five people who then control five others. This is another way logical strategy narrowed how many relationships people were oriented towards. What they did not know was that mammals who are isolated "show wild swings of unpredictable violence incompatible with membership in a social group."[3] So their tactics to counter the "savagery" they judged elsewhere actually created new types of violence. The violence of another type of competition, for me to win, you must lose. "Humans are unique because we compete when it isn't necessary. We could reason our way to more sustainable processes, but we use our intelligence to outsmart each other. We compete for fun, for ego."[9]

Without the security of the clans, this competition made families competitors. Each family unit had to provide for themselves housing, clothing and food. The family was a unit that consisted of one monogamous couple made up of one person with testicles and another person with ovaries and the biological children of that couple. Gender binaries become important in clarifying roles in making the family unit efficient and useful. When Protestantism rose in popularity, it brought more opportunity to outcompete through good work ethic. Good work ethic meant being willing and able to work harder, longer and generally more. Families compete against other families, making the family a business that produces for the marketplace where their work ethic will be judged, rewarded or punished.

To dive a bit deeply into families as businesses, let's observe the household. Families live in households. Households within the world economy are structures where the individuals within it pool income to support the household and to "share in the consumption of the income."[10] Immanuel Wallerstein outlines five types of income that can be brought into the household. Wage-income, which has been considered the "bread-winner," like going out and being paid for labor outside of the home and is considered masculine. Subsistence activity, which can be labor that produces for the household what does not need to be purchased outside the home or outsourced, like farming for your family but not to sell but also like cooking and cleaning; these are considered feminine. Petty-commodity is work that can go for sale but is not reliable, like wages. Interestingly enough, when Wallerstein describes this, he likens it to the paperboy route or selling cigarettes, things young people engage in for a quick buck or associated with poorer places, but currently, that is the gig economy and freelancing which is how many people make money under capitalism now. The fourth is rent, which is having someone else pay to live in your building or making money through investments. Money that happens without ongoing labor. Finally, there are transfer payments, which can be inheritance or money "owed," like social security. Inheritance can be the role of the elders. These ways of generating income make households and families a business.

Jeopardizing the ability of the family to make money is enough to be removed or to leave. Some contemporary examples include an elderly parent who requires care that takes time from the other adult's ability to work may be sent to a nursing home. Or an adult child who realizes their family does not compete well in the world economy may decide to leave and reject their family so they have a better chance of competing. Think here of all the movies of people leaving their families and small towns so they can go to college and move to some big city and recreate themselves. It is also a family asking their child to keep their sexuality a secret or being kicked out of their home so they will not lose credibility in their community.

Nuclear family units make some people insiders and some people outsiders. It makes a conceptual but not actual lifelong commitment to the insiders and makes the outsiders disposable or threats. Lifelong commitments are made only to spouses, children and parents. As our cultural evolution progresses, we are seeing how even these commitments are also becoming disposable, as the examples above demonstrate. This inside/outside committed/disposable paradigm translates into many aspects of life. In the West, almost everything is disposable. Our water bottles, our food, our attention. And the constant stress of being disposable to a species that needs connection and belonging makes you work hard to stay within the inside group.

Centuries later, as large governments were taking place, the message was pushed out to the masses that they should see "the Nation as Family."[4] A nation is created by preaching that you are a nation. Nation is all about making an inside and outside.[10] The goal is that adults and their children become committed not only towards their nuclear family but towards the concept of a nation. The children of the nation belong to the government and childhood becomes this important period *entrusted* to parents. Raising children becomes work and a duty to the state. This painful shift makes caregiving "unsustainable work, the massive unpaid labor that breaks backs, hearts."[5] Childhood became important because the new field of bio-power realized they were losing many potential future laborers to early death and, with those deaths went potential for profit. "For the child is regarded as the parents' property in the same way as the citizens of a totalitarian state are considered the property of its government."[11] In early Christian directives, the focus was on having the correct number of children; with the new future-oriented cultural stance, the directive was to manage these children to ensure they made it to adulthood. The family becomes the system responsible for their children to learn the rules and expectations to belong to society. Through these strategic shifts, childhood is now seen as a time where a young person is moldable and must be made submissive and they are always oriented towards a potential future.

To fulfill these new directives, sex becomes a mechanism only for reproduction, not for pleasure and not for social interaction. "Therefore, cisheterosexual sex itself becomes a means of productivity because it is understood to ultimately lead to marriage, procreation, and nuclear families, all of which are integral to patriarchal and white supremacist capitalist systems."[12] Sex becomes something hidden. This shifts the living quarters of families, introducing private bedrooms.

Parents are expected to sleep together and in rooms separate from their children. This removes children from their parents but also creates a veil of secrecy. All this secrecy of the parental bedroom later becomes the obsession of many of our favorite philosophers and early psychologists, who inform the field still to this day.

As the Industrial Revolution takes work out of the home,[3] parents are asked to be away from their children more and more but are still responsible for their outcome. Without the support of collective care or the finances to pay for care, schools become the primary forming ground for children while parents work. Schools, armies and religious and medical institutions are secondary for parents to teach children the rules they are supposed to abide by to become good and pro-ductive (see valuable) society members.[10] Good society members are individuals that self-regulate, are disciplined, independent and ambitious with a loyalty to the state. Of course, in this culture of hypocrisy and contradictions, not all fami-lies had to follow these rules. Race and wealth could help a family get around those norms. Families could have other proxies, such as the labor of people they enslaved or hired as caretakers.

In the early mid-19th century, we saw child rearing turn towards the goal of having a child that "plays well,"[4] although that sounds friendlier than crushing them into submission, the idea is still to mold them into someone other people want around. Then, in the late 20th century, "parent-child relations came to be seen as 'loving.'"[1]

These family units we have created can never successfully achieve all of the mandates placed on it. Be alone, be hard working, make a living that affords your family and all of its needs, raise children to also become hardworking and innovative because our society is relying on your child. That is a lot of pressure, and no support. We love the idea in this culture of "children are the future." We put a lot of hope, dreams and pressure on our children to materialize some unseen potential, to complete the aspirations of their parents, schools, our cul-tural groups and the nation. There is this underlying message that children are a strategy to fix something later that is broken now. Sometimes, that includes ourselves. We are culturally obsessed with finding romantic, heteronormative monogamous love in hopes it will "complete us." Or having a child because they will "complete us." I'd argue that that incomplete feeling is a symptom of society necessitating our disconnection from ourselves.

This cultural evolutionary tale looks to the family to fulfill the belonging and connection of kinship, but it fails over and over in this society because it is stra-tegic and neocortical led, not present and limbic.

More Than Machines

Today, to keep up with the mandates placed on the nuclear family, training chil-dren is an important part of parenting. "Oppression and forcing of submission do not begin in the office, factory or political party; they begin in the very first weeks of an infant's life."[11] In the West, we begin their lives by putting infants on a number of schedules (recall chrononormativity). Schedules that dictate when they should eat, sleep or be held. Later, there is potty training amongst many other trainings about controlling the body. Training children has become the optimal way of parenting. The rationality is that it prepares a child to function in the world where things are generally structured and scheduled, and by preparing the child, it increases the chances the child will compete well enough to make good money so they can live a good life, that is success.[9] And all of that is true, but the anti-oppressive question to ask here is, "Why do we want our children to succeed in this type of world?"

There is also a necessity for training children because, in our culture, caregivers are either pairs or individuals who are on schedules themselves. In New York, daycares will take infants as young as six weeks, since the US government provides no net for new parents, so parents return to work early, relative to other countries. So if a facility has multiple infants, and other children of varying ages, it's strategic to have all the children trained to eat at the same time and rest at the same time. It allows for them to give the care all the children need. This also prepares children for school. This is not the fault of the parent or the daycare. In the West, you must earn your living. In the US, there is no legal maximum of hours a person can work (and there are in other countries, by the way). The average American work week was 47 hours in 2014, and in 2018, surveys showed Americans worked 12 hours a day, and the hours keep creeping up.[13] This is not including how blurry the home and work lines have become since the COVID-19 lockdown, which made working from home a regular and expected occurrence. With adults working to provide for themselves and their nuclear families, daycares are the best options in a kinshipless culture.

This would be fine if we were, in fact, the machines our society has needed us to believe we are, but we aren't.

Some of what I will present next will seem naturally occurring (which I hope by now sets off your alarms). However, the structures of brains of highly literate cultures are different from those that are not.[8] Most of those differences take place in the neocortex, our analytic brain, and may not rule out that the limbic brain has more qualities that are experienced in other humans across cultures.

When a human infant leaves the womb, they are more likely to respond when hearing the voice of their birthing parent than anyone else. If that parent speaks a native language, they have more pleasure hearing the native language.[3] Why is that? Because from in utero, a child's social engagement system is active. This is implicit, an awareness that comes from the senses. "At this point there is no personality, no filtering, and no social conditioning, just the basic movement of the conscious awareness as it comes into the relational field of the family and the world."[7]

The social engagement system of a human is activated 24 to 28 weeks in gestation, unlike the rest of the motor skills that may take up to years to develop.[14] This system develops with the limbic brain. The system activates the muscles around the head and face, throat, middle ear and voice box so that the infant can signal to caregivers of its needs as soon as they are birthed onto the planet. For human babies, like many other species of newborns, going to their nourishment is unavailable, so we tune into the social engagement system. This system brings nourishment to the infant. Here, remember an example of a parent who knows that one quality of crying from their babies means they are hungry, and that motivates the parent to bring food, and they can distinguish it from another cry that means they have had an excretion and the parents must go clean the infant. Human babies are prepared to come out into the world and communicate with their caregivers their needs, and there is a flurry of hormones in a birthing parent that prepares them to meet the needs of their infant, who cannot speak and ask. Here, they utilize limbic attunement or resonance.

Recall here that feminized traits (limbic qualities) such as nurturing, tenderness, protection, receptivity and perception most associated with birthing parents are undervalued in this society. Those limbic qualities flow freely in societies oriented towards connectivity, a limbic resonant society. In Japan, there is an emotion called amae. English does not have an emotional equivalent, so I will describe it. Amae is basically the type of attention towards a young person who isn't expected to do anything but what they are moved to and must be supported by those around them.[1] Societal expectations dictate emotions. In ours, amae would be something we consider spoiled, unrealistic or setting the child up to fail as an adult because, in our culture, it is unrealistic to believe you can have your needs reflected and met, make mistakes and still belong. We could never do amae here because, in Japan, amae is part of the development of a well-rounded person who can understand how to respond to amae because they have had it. It is a cultural value to maintain connection. The culture encourages this as an acceptable and admirable way of being. Here in the United States specifically, when parents attempt to replicate this way of child raising without a real understanding of how culture informs everything, it will not yield the same results. We live in a violent and individualist society where the child will be oriented towards getting their own needs met, not that of another, and may lead to more self-centeredness rather than the attention to others it leads to in Japan.

This is one example of how feelings are responsive to a culture. Think about how often you speak to someone from another country who speaks another language, and they want to express a feeling or experience, and they say there is not a direct English translation, so they proceed to describe it using many English words. That is because their culture allows for those feelings.

Westerners see emotions as separate from the body, from relationships, that they too are inside of us and private. We believe that they originate from deep places in us and not around us. That seems true here because it has been made to be true. It is not true everywhere and often not really true of us either. Emotions are created within context. Social connection, the context that emotions are in, is more important to the wellbeing of human development than food, water and shelter.[15] And that's been proven time and time again. Failure to Thrive refers to a series of unrelated studies that found that even if a human infant has all their physiological needs met yet is deprived of physical touch and affection from caregivers; the infant will struggle physically and, in many cases, die.[3] Since our orientation is towards living long and productive lives, this is devastating.

This is possible because the limbic brain takes in a lot of information about the environment and what then our bodies should do in response. Polyvagal theory, although complicated, is ultimately about how our nervous system communicates from the brain to the body in response to input from the environment. This mammalian system uses all parts of the brain and gut. When an infant first perceives danger, they first activate the social engagement system; this may be the crying, yelling, wincing of the face. If that does not alleviate the threat, we may see them activate the sympathetic nervous system, bringing in our oldest brain, which connects to the heart and lungs, preparing us to fight or flight. If all else fails, the system goes to shutdown, impacting the stomach, kidneys, and intestines.[16] Danger can be a bear attack, but it can also be the subtle emotional shift in the room or a threat of disconnection from others.

The care expressed through connection or reflecting literally creates an environment that signals safety and belonging; it regulates the baby's heart, digestive system and motivates cell growth. Using the limbic system, infants and young children respond to the emotional and nervous systems of their caregivers and use them to regulate their own inner states.[4] Feeling cared for is not internal; it is an external experience. You could whisper softly to a baby all day that you love them from a few feet away; they still will die from lack of that care expressed in a way that reaches *how they need it*, and they will not have an innate sense of being cared for. "Feelings are critical measures of one's condition."[17] Emotions are not inside of us; they are between us.[1] "Successful synchrony between two mammals is an acrobatic maneuver wherein each catches another's rhythms and adjusts his own accordingly."[4] Within 30 minutes of isolation, cortisol, the body's stress hormone, inflates six times its original levels.[3] Being able to attune to and adjust based on the needs of another being is mammalian and is happening with or without our awareness.

Feel Into It

How do you *feel* (not think) about feelings being something that occurs between not inside? How is your inside responding to this external stimulus?

Practice to Intervention

What do we do with the narrative "no one has the power to make you feel anything"? It's pervasive and untrue. Our feelings are based on an external world. What does it mean to accept that an external experience did make us feel something? Try using this lens for some time. Notice what curiosities arose when doing so. Share your observations with your group.

However, through training, we teach infants that bodies are to be regulated and having needs met is earned. Because in white, middle-class American families (our ideal), the goal is to become independent.[1] I know as psychotherapists, we are familiar with the failure to thrive concept; however, we still do support parents to train their children away from connection. We are still writing articles and blogs about it, running parenting programs emphasizing raising independent children. This is the cognitive dissonance our industry is seeped in.

We teach that discipline and self-regulation are preferred. We teach a baby not only with words but with our ability to limbically resonate. For example, let's say a parent is trying to sleep train their baby (because, remember, here we place babies in separate rooms from their parents); although the baby may cry for a long time, the parent will stay away, ignoring even their own longing to soothe their baby. This is what I mean about training away from the body. The parent is also undergoing the training of going against their instinct and hormonal charge to rescue their baby for the ideals of the society that an independent baby is going to be a successful baby. Already, we are instilling the value that a body that is apologetic about having needs, desires, and wants is a preferred body.

The way we as people apologize for having needs is by having discipline, being orderly and polite, even if everything in our body says, "THIS IS NOT RIGHT!" We teach our children not to trust their feelings or the cues of their bodies, to trust authorities instead, that they know better about what the child needs. This is where a child learns to ignore "their gut feelings and in numbing awareness . . . learn to hide from their selves."[16] Without the limbic resonance that responds to and validates the bodily needs of an infant, they cannot sense how to use their own limbic systems and will have difficulty identifying themselves.[3] This indoctrinates the child to "self-objectification," the belief that our bodies are something we can control and use with our minds, which is separate from ourselves.[13] I have not heard of another animal that can think it is separate from its body. But they probably exist somewhere out there.

Here is an example of a system wired towards resonating and connection. I realized my limbic attunement to others was still very active even when I'm unaware, my first weekend in Hakomi year 1. We were learning about the skill called tracking, which I now interpret as activating our limbic systems to notice another's. As I was learning about that, I realized I am always tracking without awareness. For example, I am cooking with a friend and we are engaged in conversation as we prepare our food. They turn to me and ask, "Did I already put salt in this?" I take a few seconds trying to recall using explicit memory if I saw it or not, but I cannot recall because I was engaged in conversation. But when they ask me, "Did you see where I put my glasses?" I point without thinking. Somehow, I was noticing my friend and tracking my friend but not with any awareness. I did not remember noticing them put their glasses down, but I was somehow quite aware of how to find them.

Explicit memory is what we think is useful to store. We are cooking so, obviously, what I should have been tracking is our meal preparation and the salt, but my limbic memory is tracking the relational field and has its own priorities. I was tracking what was important to my friend despite the neocortical task at hand. Tracking is not intuition, but it orients us towards being receptive and having agendaless curiosity. Whether we are noticing it or not, we are tracking, and what we track can be recalled implicitly. Implicit memory is memory stored through sensing. Lewis, Amini and Lannon share an anecdote about a study participant who had amnesia, loss of storing new explicit memory, but was taught how to braid.[4] Every time he was asked if he knew how to braid, he would say no, but if you put some string in front of him, he would braid it. This is an example of his explicit memory never storing that he learned how to braid but the senses, implicit memory, remember the action. That is limbic magic!

Practice to Intervention

Do you know this experience? A time when you are noticing things that seem insignificant and, later on, they happen to be very significant? What did you call that then? What is it like recalling it now?

Start noticing what you notice. We are trained away from noticing in this culture, instead prioritizing focus. But what we notice as clinicians is an intervention in itself. Increasing this ability through practice is an important exercise in widening our view.

Let us return to our sleep-trained infant. So, when that baby subdues from their crying, that is the social engagement system rewiring. The baby now limbically understands that the world will not give them what they need. Because the social engagement system does not only bring to an infant what they need, it also brings the infant into a community. It is the system that learns to smile when others smile and supports a sense of safety by tuning into the beings around them. The infant is learning through their limbic system and the reptilian brain about how they should be to have their needs met and to belong. The child is also creating implicit memories in the body, since the neocortical brain has yet to fully develop. So, by the time we explicitly tell the child they need to work hard, they have already implicitly stored that information from their preverbal experiences.

Limbic disconnection is not that the limbic system stops doing what it is doing; it stops expecting a response, to be met or to be welcomed. So, as the neocortex develops, the child can rely on this barely developed brain to protect and hide their limbic system from the pain of being unmet. The child creates a strategy before their strategic brain is fully developed. The purpose of this strategy is not understood by the neocortex; it is stored in the body and is oriented to staying connected.

The modern Western child, especially if they are living in a city, is feeling a lack of belonging in their human connections because the limbic system is also lacking belonging to an environment that includes non-human beings. Prior to electricity and the ability to extend days into nights or housing that was not on the ground or completely enclosed off from the surrounding topography – infants' senses were attuned to nature as well as their caregivers. With a culture moving away from being part of or being nature, infant humans are responding more and more to the overstimulation of artificial sounds, lights, smells, textures and tastes.[18] Our worlds are so controlled that there is very little space for surprise, discovery, delight and it is simply about plugging into the rhythm already set in motion. Our senses, in many ways, "have been stripped."[4] Not only the ones we think of like taste, sight, sound, hearing, but our sense of intuition and connection to land and spirit. The overfocusing on training children also limits the possibilities of their senses. If we only believe the child can or should be crying for a certain amount of things, like food, diaper change or tired, we are unaware that we are only focused on their training, not on what they are possible of. I wonder what it would be like to recognize a child's cry that communicates "I need sunlight," or "I want to hear someone's voice," or "the Earth is in pain" or the many other possibilities my limited brain cannot imagine.

Practice to Intervention

Meditation can re-engage these senses and maintain their engagement longer term, but so can other orgiastic states, including psychedelics. These medicines, substances and drugs impact the limbic system and can support our ability to integrate the outside world senses with what we feel within, which is a whole different sense on its own.[19] This is all a part of re-relating to oneself through feeling one's needs and the response of the environment. This may include a sense of a world in pain, a sense of animals in pain, a sense of the Earth crying etc. These are real senses people can experience when in expanded states. However, in this culture, these experiences may be dismissed as unimportant or pathologized. My colleague and friend Bill Brennan warns that our usual tactics often "take an experience about a large-scale injustice and make it about the patient."[20] We may do this instead of recognizing that, actually, more of their senses are available to them, so are their connections to themselves and their surroundings.

Think this has relevance in your practice? With yourself? With the people you serve?

Creating a Good Individual

Thus is the plight of a Western child. The abandonment of attunement is not done out of cruelty; it is to be replaced by what the caregivers in the environment believe will be more useful in surviving in this collective. And these caregivers are right. A culture that says sacrificing personal needs for potential future gains is impressive because once we achieve such greatness, we will finally be deserving of safety and ease.[13] We are increasing other parts of the brain while downplaying the importance of this mammalian superpower.[8] What we are increasing is our neocortical brain, the brain that analyzes, the brain that innovates, strategizes what is logical and strives for reason. We are increasing the need to have a persona, a personality that will get us what we need. This split increases the dissonance between a public and a private sense of self. The private now includes the emotional body and bodily needs. This concept of emotions being something internal and separate is a very Western idea. The global majority understand emotions as something "public, social and relational."[1] In these majority settings where emotions are seen as acts between people, there is not a concept of some emotions being more natural than others; the emotion is responsive to the relationship and the context. The developmental models that come out of the psychological sciences reinforce that some feelings are natural and appropriate while others are not. But "development is much messier than our logical, reconstructive theories would have us believe."[21]

So we "develop the art of performing in order to get the love we need."[22] Certain ways of being are unacceptable, and we must hide them. This is the same internalization of norms that led to the creation of a private self described in Chapter 3. Remember, by suppressing the unacceptable, we are fragmenting ourselves; we create in ourselves a private part and we cultivate a public performance. Our public performance should always be striving, and if we are not striving it will indicate that we are always "slothful or unaccomplished" because of attribution error.[13] As we recall from Chapter 3, this was the reason many individuals were admitted to early hospitals for being lazy. Ambition should be in our public performance even now and in friendship.

From childhood, we encourage children to create personalities that will attract friends. Due to fundamental attribution error, we expect that personality to be the same regardless of the circumstance. In many cultures, making "personal adjustments to differing relationships" is seen as "reflecting wisdom, maturity, and social adeptness" as opposed to in America, where it is registered as "two-face"[8] or "people pleasing," which are both major insults in the West.

All young mammals play. Play is an important part of locating the self in relationship to others. However, how we treat making friends in the West is less about free play and more about skill building and learning to "play well with others." Making friends is the childhood version of voluntary organizations. Striving for peer acceptance is seen as a normal part of child development but what it begins to cultivate is an orientation towards status.[4] These voluntary associations, like the adult ones, do not have our best interest at heart since they are trying to have their needs met too. These peer groups are a bunch of children who, like us, are looking to be accepted and belong. And all of us in the group learned love is conditional and acceptance is earned. This is already happening in the home, in the school and being reinforced in these playgroups. This is still teaching children that become adults "to achieve, not attach."[3] In many cultures, making friends is more trouble than they are worth. In our culture, we are trained towards finding like-mindedness, to abandon our families that do not think like us, which leads us to search for a chosen family. Listen, chosen families save lives. This is not a dig at that, but there is a certain kind of grief I feel that we expect to not be accepted by kin and forced to make kin. That grief is not about an individual having to find a chosen family; it's about the conditions that make it a necessity.

Rob Brezny, an eccentric astrologer I follow, once quoted Carolyn Godschild Miller in one of his emails where she asks, "Why is it so hard to find a soulmate?" And she responds to her own question with this:

Because most of us are actually searching for egomates instead. We place the most limited and unloving aspect of our minds in charge of our search for love, and then wonder why we aren't succeeding. To the degree that we identify with this false sense of self, and operate on the basis of its limited point of view, we aren't looking for someone to love so much as recruiting fellow actors to take on supporting roles in a favorite melodrama.[23]

I do not know how much she thinks about performance and backstage, but we are reading from the same script here. We are looking to fill limbic needs with neocortical strategies. Consider what this means for therapy. Many of the more popular and mainstream theories and methods continue to enroll the neocortex, hoping it will finally figure out how to fill the limbic gap. We cannot talk, think, behave our way into healing these absences that are often preverbal wounds and later conditioned to stay away. So much energy goes into sustaining our performances. What good limbic resonance can do is signal to the brain, "No need to perform here; both the backstage and front stage can co-exist" or "I am not invested in parts of you; I am interested in you as you are with me now." That is acceptance. That's what is missing when we train our children towards fragmentation.

An Ego Deserving of Love

Some emotions are good, and they are rewarded to make them habits. We sustain those habits because we limbically understand love is conditional. One of the good emotions is love. Naturally, "love is an invention of societies that are organized around autonomous individuals; it is needed less in societies where relationship networks are unquestioned and permanent."[1] In kinship-based networks, what we may call love that can appear as care, affection, closeness is freely given. But in the West, none of our relationships are unquestioned and meant to be permanent. The sense that they can suddenly end compels us to create egos and performances deserving of love. And the standards for what is deserving are high. We will go into the proper emotions in a second, but there are deserving physical appearances; love in the West has so much to do with "whether or not others locate desire in you."[24] Whether your physical body is desirable and then whether it is usable. In many ways, we see the body as a barrier to receiving love, something to overcome to get love. Due to this conditioning, we ignore that the body is actually the home of our sense of emotions; the names and values we assign those emotions, that's from the mind.[25] Since not all emotions are acceptable, we must disconnect from the body or become disembodied.[25] This disembodiment strengthens the pathway that understands the body can be objectified, used to attract love or at least to work and prove we deserve love. We have to perform active bodies because lazy bodies definitely do not deserve love.[13]

Feel Into It

Pause here. Feel here. Love isn't a feeling where relationships are permanent. What is stirred in you? Does it make you want to express yourself in some way? Let that happen. Check on your jaw, chest/back, glutes and hips.

"You can get a semblance of love or acceptance for being polite or unburdensome," we train this in our children, who are socialized as women. We ask that they store away unpleasant emotions and perform being nice and unbothersome; this will keep people around. We shut down the vulnerability necessary for limbic resonance in exchange for pleasantness. Although multiple studies now show that certain chronic illnesses have a strong link to the suppression of anger in exchange for politeness.[4] To the point that doctors could guess accurately the diagnosis of a patient based on the disposition of the patient. The polite, unburdensome, repressing self to avoid conflict or for others, comfort personality types were more likely to get chronic illness, and their diagnoses were more fatal.[4]

For our conditioning of man children, they get love by performing dominance, power over others and themselves; we can see this in anger. This comes with its own set of diseases.

The suppression of vulnerable emotions, of course, is one manifestation of male-trauma, leading inexorably to a withering of compassion for others – especially when those others have something we want, as in every instance of date rape or nonconsensual sexual aggression.[4]

These are more social diseases we all suffer from. Testosterone does increase aggression, so there is a hormonal component, but we cannot blame that because, as we've already covered, culture and child-rearing can override genetics. Testicles and testosterone are not exclusive to the West, and in other cultures, the type of aggression displayed from Western people is viewed as demonic.[4]

Even though babies are giving us signals from the moment they come out to the world, we have ones we prefer. We love when they make faces that look like smiling or when they seem to laugh. We want all of our children and our adults to perform happiness. Happiness in the US is about "feeling good about yourself"[1] and is seen as the optimal state of being rather than the fleeting emotion it actually is. Feeling good about yourself and being proud is healthy here. Having pride, having self-esteem are signs of happiness, so is feeling superior. And if you do not feel these ways, something may be wrong.

Gosh, we therapists collude so hard here. I know I have and still do feel the pressure to help my clients feel happy or proud of themselves. We judge and blame parents who produce children with "low self-esteem" because they make them feel shame.

In this culture, shame is unacceptable.[8] Because shame is like a painful admission that other people's experience of you matters, and we see "relying on other people as a threat to progress."[13] And yet, in many cultures, shame is what keeps people committed to relationships, to their kin. It is an honorable emotion, not disgraceful or painful. Being boastful can be disgraceful in other cultures and is celebrated here. Shame signals you have not met an expectation of the community, and feeling and expressing shame is how you emote that you want to stay connected, aren't looking to be in a power position and willing to be held accountable. Competence is the opposite; it's like putting on our power-up suit; it's our shield, protection from shame.

I think this is so important for therapists who must often prove how competent we are, and since no one else is in the room with us and the client, how we speak about our work is used to evaluate our competence. Avoiding shame and accountability may create the conditions for inaccurate tellings of our work. Even within the session, it's hard to allow shame to take up space when it is present in the client or in the therapy room if we are working hard to avoid our own shame. And, to combat shame, we strive to perform more competence or perfection. Because competence and confidence are good, they demonstrate our individual greatness, while shame is bad because it is connected to others seeing our not greatness. Dr. Joy Degruy has this heartbreaking example she shares of how, for the enslaved person, increasing shame in their child was a survival tactic. The less competent their child seemed, the less likely they would be taken and separated from their parent. This adaptation has continued and can be seen today in Black families.[26] This makes Black children less successful in a world that rewards lack of shame.

Our strategic neocortex is like, "Oh, you want to never feel shame? No problem. I will never let you see anything that will make you feel shameful." That's cognitive dissonance. It creates entire illusions for us, which is easy to do because we stopped trusting our bodies a long time ago to feel things out. This level of cognitive dissonance produces a culture that is quite superficial, avoidant and fragile. In an individual, this could look like an out-of-touch, grandiose person. In this culture, we reward grandiosity and unintentionally train children towards it.

However, "the grandiose person is never really free; first, because he is excessively dependent on admiration from others, and second, because his self-respect is dependent on qualities, functions and achievements that can suddenly fail."[11] Along with the grandiosity comes a set of entitlements and individual rights that need protecting (recall rights being made up to control). Between the disembodiment, the shield of competence, the superficiality, avoidance, protection of entitlements and fragility, a culture organized around these sentiments can never be communal. Communal in other cultures and historically meant relational harmony was where all the energy goes. But all of our energy is linked to protecting the self. And more also, we admire competent, rights-protecting, angry yet pleasant people; those are our leaders, they are who we give power to. These ways of being are what maintain our swan dive towards the sixth mass extinction. "Our wounded leaders with their blinkered priorities enact social policies that keep conditions how they were, or worse."[4] When I say grandiosity, I am not only thinking of who we perceive as our classic narcissistic leader but also our martyrs who believe their pain and experiences are some big offering to the planet or society, or the hopeless that believe the whole world is conspiring against them. Can you think of other ways to queer grandiosity?

Thanissara warns that

we should not be misled by our human hubris and assume we will secure our future, that in some magical way we deserve to be here on this magnificent planet and that it is our inborn right to always use her resources.[7]

But her warning, I fear, is a bit late.

Our entitlement and grandiosity are fragile. It also skews our view of what we "deserve" in the world and how to get it. Our beliefs about what we deserve and the lack of those experiences increase isolation and loneliness. "Because we are biopsychosocial creatures, the rising loneliness epidemic in Western culture is much more than just a psychological phenomenon; it is a public health crisis" Maté writes.[4] Mia Birdsong shares the findings of a 2018 survey that found that one in four Americans felt they had no one in their lives who understood them. She goes on to share that 43% felt that they always lacked companionship, had no meaningful relationships and were isolated from others.[15] And the cultural belief that we must work to alleviate our own suffering (aka the Protestant work ethic) increases suicide. Statistical analysis of 19th-century Prussia shows that Protestant countries had about 15 more suicides per 100,000 people.[8]

Although I am highlighting how these preferred ways of being are anti-collective, it is a privilege in this culture to be raised this way. We must remember not all Western children get this upbringing. The oppressive system we inhabit is not made for everyone to have the "privilege of being an individual." When care may be present, but pride is not, think of immigrant families that utilize shame to keep kinship strong. People in these systems will work hard to please their family members and exhibit what we would call "low self-esteem," if they come to therapy, we may create goals for them to only care about themselves and to be proud of themselves. When care may be present but physical needs are unmet, think of people who are taken from their families through child protective services or people who are made poor through our culture's economy based on profit over everything. These people may not see the need to perform pleasant-ness or politeness because they see how unpleasant life really is, but in therapy, we might gaslight them into thinking their view of the world is the issue and a kinder view would allow for kinder experiences. When care may be present but competence is not, think of those we discount for having any social value due to perceived or real ability; they may depend on others. We in therapy might try to make them more independent, so they do not have to rely on their loved ones. These are examples of how therapy often is used to break up some of the kin-based connections that exist in exchange for normal and good individuals.

Feel Into It

How do you feel shame in your body? What tells you? Really sit with that for as long as you can.

Who can you talk to about what has come up? Is there shame here?

Practice to Intervention

How do you react to other people's shame?

I know some clinicians, theories and methods who do not have a power analysis and enjoy their seat as an authority who use shame as a motivator to move clients' change in a direction they feel is suitable. They may even increase shame to get the client in a state of willingness to change. This is not the suggestion of this writer. Because the client and therapist are not kin. That is an abuse of power.

I know, for myself as someone in the therapist's seat that is very mindful of the power I yield, I tend to avoid shame. Afraid of either using the combination of shame and power to influence like those I named above or because I am uncomfortable with my own shame. This fear of shame is also not the recommendation of this book.

I remember with RL how often I tried to negate their shame. But their drug usage did isolate people from them. It did make life harder. I now believe if I stayed with the shame, let it fully be felt, expressed and present instead of trying to shoo it away, we would have gotten to some grief and pain. I imagine that the grief and pain would have been present because those people, this society who made RL feel shame, were not attached or committed to RL. They were not invested in getting RL back into the relationship and they were not willing to shift for them either.

That's the thing with shame in an idealized connected community. The community also is committed to getting you back in good standing, it is also going to shift so that you can. Unlike here, where shame is about a personal failure, and you are left to figure it out on your own, and as a consequence of your behavior and the community will not adjust to meet you.

How will you increase your tolerance to neither avoid nor use shame but to allow it in the client and in the space? How will you increase your tolerance of shame in yourself?

We Are Unwell

As a culture, we are obsessed with health- but what is making us most "unhealthy" is our culture that has evolved to sever co-regulating and affirming kin while breeding entitled individuals. And the professions created to dictate health ignore this. "The prevailing medical paradigm has no capacity to incorporate the concept that a relationship is a physiological process, as real and as potent as any pill or surgical procedure."[3] Our detachment from our bodies, spirit and land do not help. What is making us unhealthy is the isolation necessary to succeed in this culture. "Another way of saying it: chronic illness-mental or physical- is to a large extent a *function* or *feature* of the way things are and not a *glitch*; a consequence of how we live, not a mysterious aberration."[4]

"If trauma entails a disconnection from the self, then it makes sense to say that we are being collectively flooded with influences that both exploit and reinforce trauma."[4] People are going into therapy every day for an array of reasons and, often, it dwindles down to them wanting to express themselves and still belong at work, home, in their relationships whether romantic, familial, platonic, sexual, etc. Often, not even knowing what they would want to express if they could do so freely. This is an old wound, but it's not an individual wound. It is a historical and cultural wound. Desire to belong, to be interdependent is not immature and does not go away as we age. As clinicians, I believe it is our duty to remember our own longings for interdependence, to grieve the disappointments of not having it so that we can always have it in our awareness when working with others. In this culture, our minds, bodies and souls are deeply malnourished.[4]

What we will need to take with us on this journey forward is that social connection and a sense of belonging are vital to the wellbeing of mammals, not optional. It really will take some unlearning to divest from the hierarchy of needs as we have been taught. These false understandings of how human life is organized seeps into everything, our self-talk, parenting, education, spirituality, relationships, politics, social support systems, housing and the list goes on and on. We need to see how insidious it is in ourselves, in our culture and in our profession so we can divest from it and open ourselves up to the vulnerability and the possibilities that come with it.

Feel Into It

Let the dust settle.

Citations

1. Mesquita, B. (2022). *Between us: How cultures create emotions.* W. W. Norton & Company.
2. Haraway, D. J. (2016). *Staying with the trouble: Making Kin in the Chthulucene (experimental futures)* (Illustrated). Duke University Press Books.
3. Lewis, T., Amini, F., & Lannon, R. (2001). *A general theory of love* (Reprint). Vintage.
4. Maté, G., MD, & Maté, D. (2022). *The myth of normal: Trauma, illness, and healing in a toxic culture.* Avery.
5. Gumbs, A. P., & Brown, A. M. (2020). *Undrowned: Black feminist lessons from marine mammals (emergent strategy, 2).* AK Press.
6. Haden, P., Middleton, D., & Robinson, P. (1995). A historical and critical essay for Black women. In B. Guy-Sheftall (Ed.), *Words of fire: An anthology of African American feminist thought.* The New Press.
7. Thanissara. (2015). *Time to stand up: An engaged Buddhist manifesto for our earth -- The Buddha's life and message through feminine eyes (sacred activism)* (1st ed.). North Atlantic Books.
8. Henrich, J. (2021). *WEIRDest people in the world: How the west became psychologically peculiar and particularly prosperous.* Picador Paper.
9. Brown, A. M. (2019). *Pleasure activism: The politics of feeling good.* AK Press.
10. Wallerstein, I. (2004). World-systems analysis. In *Duke University Press eBooks.* Duke University Press. https://doi.org/10.1215/9780822399018

11. Miller, A. (1997). *The drama of the gifted child: The search for the true self* (revised ed., 3rd ed.). Basic Books.
12. Brown, S. (2022). *Refusing compulsory sexuality: A Black asexual lens on our sex-obsessed culture*. North Atlantic Books.
13. Price, D., PhD. (2022). *Laziness does not exist*. Atria.
14. Porges, S. W. (2006). The role of social engagement in attachment and bonding: A phylogenetic perspective. In *Attachment and bonding: A new synthesis* (pp. 33–54). The MIT Press. ISBN: 0-262-03348-8
15. Birdsong, M. (2020). *How we show up: Reclaiming family, friendship, and community*. Hachette Go.
16. Kolk, V. B. der, MD. (2015). *The body keeps the score: Brain, mind, and body in the healing of trauma* (Reprint). Penguin Publishing Group.
17. Leiner, R., & Syedullah, J. (2023). The manual for liberating survival: Lesson I, how self-care matters as an embodied practice of abolition. In A. Crawley & R. Sirvent (Eds.), *Spirituality and abolition*. Common Notions.
18. Louv, R. (2006). *Last child in the woods: Saving our children from nature-deficit disorder*. Algonquin Books.
19. Tafur, J., MD. (2017). *The fellowship of the river: A medical doctor's exploration into traditional Amazonian plant medicine*. Espiritu Books.
20. Brennan, B. P. (2020, August 11). *The revolution will not be psychologized: Psychedelics' potential for systemic change*. Chacruna. https://chacruna.net/the-revolution-will-not-be-psychologized-psychedelics-potential-for-systemic-change/
21. Johanson, G. (2015). Hakomi principles and a systems approach to psychotherapy. In H. Weiss, L. Monda, & G. Johanson (Eds.), *Hakomi mindfulness-centered somatic psychotherapy: A comprehensive guide to theory and practice* (1st ed.). W.W. Norton & Company, Inc.
22. Williams, A. K., Owens, R., & Syedullah, J., PhD. (2016). *Radical dharma: Talking race, love, and liberation* (Illustrated). North Atlantic Books.
23. Brezsny, R. (2022, February 8). *Relationships need artful imagination*. https://news letter.freewillastrology.com/p/relationships-need-artful-imagination
24. Harrison, D. L., & Laymon, K. (2021). *Belly of the beast: The politics of anti-fatness as anti-blackness*. North Atlantic Books.
25. Owens, L. R. (2020). *Love and rage: The path of liberation through anger*. North Atlantic Books.
26. AJ+. (2019, November 8). Post traumatic slave syndrome. How is it different from PTSD? | AJ+ Opinion. *YouTube*. www.youtube.com/watch?v=Rorgjdvphek

Chapter 5

Personal Responsibility

Feel Into It

Take A Breath:

Start with some breathing/grounding here.
Take a moment. Find your seat.
Feel/imagine/see your body breathing.
Give yourself a few moments.
Find your seat, feel your body.
Take your time.

An Impossible Task

So far, we have skimmed the surface of social norms we take on as natural but were created in response to historical context and cultural evolution of the West. Many of these were not done intentionally but evolved out of our collective consciousness. The collective consciousness of the West being consumed with an afterlife and fear of eternal punishment for not being good changed the psychology of the West quicker than any other naturally occurring input. This fear made each individual responsible for their own morality and required these new individuals to abandon their kinship-based networks, destroying the connection to kin and land needed to feel belonging. This shifted our focus to an analytical and logical neocortex supremacy that strategizes to recreate those lost kinship connections and belonging. It is so important that all of us, psychotherapists, but especially us, who want to practice in an anti-oppressive way, study and have a sense of the cultural evolution of our society to be with the really complicated and nuanced truth of our existence. Without much insight as to how that separation occurred, we easily replicate the same actions that brought the disconnection.

DOI: 10.4324/9781003207054-7

Those beliefs are in us, and we must "recognize how we constantly enact culture in our everyday interactions."[1]

Often, client's come to us in an attempt to remedy some disconnection they are experiencing. Without having a real pulse on our collective disconnection, we are set up to send them back out on the search, colluding with the belief that what they are looking for is only elusive because of who they are and how much they are willing to work. The profession often is inadvertently (or purposefully) implying that with more sincere effort, they may find that oh-so-slippery happiness. In this culture, happiness is a sign of success and is our reward for our hard work, good health and being normal. We work towards happiness because it is supposed to bring that missing connection and belonging we are strategizing for. But most of the time, it doesn't. Because that disconnection was severed centuries ago and passed down generationally and systematically and, for most of us, it was personally severed at infancy. It disconnected us from our bodies and our limbic intelligence, which tells us where we are, who we are and what we belong to.

This impossible task of mending that disconnection through happiness dictates almost all of a Westerner's life without our awareness or consent. Which is why I critique our industry so much and the role of the therapist (more to come). And still, I cannot imagine doing anything else to survive capitalism. Us therapists get to witness the lives of fellow wanders and dream with them. We are in such a rare position to meet someone in their vulnerability and accept them as they are. We have the unusual opportunity to meet them with skillful limbic attunement. Unfortunately, on top of the cultural indoctrination we all experience, therapists are further trained to hide our vulnerability as well.

So, what does it mean to be a clinician that is practicing anti-oppression? It is to be deeply curious and concerned about how, as a profession, we have been given the responsibility to maintain an oppressive society. In Chapter 5, we get to explore just that: the role of the helper in Western society. We will dive into the professional ancestors of the psychotherapist, the doctor and the priest. Then, we will turn towards the institutions that initiate us.

Feel Into It

This is an invitation to become undone. To be suspicious of all you have not considered about why you want to do this work. To notice where you feel offended, where you feel seen, where you feel ashamed, where you feel vindicated – those often are good starting points to unravel and shed the identity of the professional helper. Share these noticings with your reading group.

The Helper

The helper in any society is guided by the commitments and priorities of the society. We have this incorrect idea that the helper helps individuals; actually, the helper helps society. In kinship-based societies the helper supports individuals or groups to stay connected. In societies committed to maintaining the connection between the seen and unseen worlds, the helper may primarily support in identifying and performing rituals. What is the role of the helper in the society we have been unfolding in the last three chapters? One that culturally evolved to prioritize scaling up, therefore, creates a commitment to order and control? What is the role of the helper in the West, a culture consumed by individual responsibility? The helper is the professional. A profession is primarily a voluntary organization with a marketplace value. Recall that joining a voluntary organization with a marketplace value is one of the neocortical strategies to feel belonging. The helping profession is an identity, a personality, a performance. The professional is always someone who works on behalf of the powerful in hopes of getting a need of theirs's met as well.

In the early stages of this scaled-up society, the helpers were priests. The consciousness of the time was to create societies that were cooperative. Cooperation was forged by being fearful of a growing god, therefore, living by the rules of the church would please this god. The people who could help individuals in their purpose of pleasing God were priests. The priest had the ability, once there was a confession of wrongdoing and wrong thought, desire or impulse, to direct the sinner towards the penance necessary to clear the slate. At first, this was exclusive to the wealthy elites, but with time, lay people could also receive this holy aid. As scaling increased in the West, consciousness, led by elites, turned towards creating perfect cities that reflected heaven on earth. This meant dealing with individuals that tarnished the aesthetic of the cities. Those that appeared to refuse to work (whether it was actual refusal or not, mattered less), those that were "mad" and those that rebelled or disagreed needed to be hidden. This created the helpers such as the police, the prison and hospital staff. The professional helper came out of these institutions.

When the values of the collective, led by governments, shifted towards being able to increase wealth and predict financial growth, these professionals became experts. "The doctor becomes the great advisor and expert, if not in the art of governing, at least in that observing, correcting and improving the social body and maintaining it in a permanent state of health."[2] These experts made individuals into cases, and those cases became data points. The individual that becomes a case is academic property. Cases have been historically and are still used in an attempt to predict an individual's value based on their lives so far. We still use this language today, like in "case presentations."[3] These experts forecast productivity and the optimal set of behaviors that would increase the length of time someone could be productive to society. These behaviors were declared healthy, normal and the sign of modern humans.

To distribute and surveil adherence to these new norms and health standards, the helpers are called out of the big cities and start building practices in small towns everywhere. These doctors, nurses, and later social welfare workers make up the systems; institutions necessary to maintain rapid growth and maximum extraction for greater society. They oversaw compliance to norms and health standards and found ways to help individuals or individual families meet the norms. These people become the eyes and ears of the government, vowing to report anyone not following the guidelines of normal. The helpers are like the semi-periphery nation-states of the world economy.[4] Remember, semi-periphery nation-states provide the labor for core nations in the hopes that they, too, can become a core state. There is a need to believe that all is equal and possible, and if we work for the state, we will have access to the benefits of state loyalty and maybe ascend out of enforcement into being in the position to dictate rules.

The role of the helper is also responsible for quieting potential disturbances and encouraging loyalty to society. We utilize two main strategies to do this. First, by reinforcing it is an individual's failure for their lot in life, and we will "out of the goodness of our hearts" help them course correct. Our second strategy is to supplement their needs. Giving the false sense of being taken care of by the government. But remember, states do not serve; they need servants. Both strategies ignore that our social context is why they are without in the first place. That clarity gets muddied when there is a whole industry purporting they are the government's response to an individual's crisis. The helper has been enrolled in this idea (especially the anti-oppressive one) that by supporting the "most marginalized," we can shift tides; the research shows us differently. In the United States, the more citizens who favor a policy change when our elite class disagrees, the less likely it will happen.[5] This democratic lie continues to misguide all of us, but us helpers really need to snap out of it because we are the backbone of the charade.

With the helper playing such a vital role in society, we must explore this role. We will specifically look at the modern psychotherapist. The modern psychotherapist, whether coming from the angle of Social Work that also includes a lean towards charity work, and/or the Case Worker, which leans more towards the police, the Psychiatrist, which leans more towards the doctor or the Psychoanalyst that leans more towards the priest. All of these roles are mixed into the psychotherapist as helper.

Psychotherapy's Ancestry: Public Performance, Private Shadow

Just a reminder that out of cultural necessity, people of the West created shadow. Shadow includes what should not be seen and must be hidden, as it will disturb the performance needed to be admitted into voluntary organizations. The largest voluntary organizations are nations. And to remain in membership of Western nations, you must perform that you have value for the marketplace. The stakes are high for individuals of the West to maintain their marketplace value since belonging is not assumed but must be earned over and over again. Humans, like other mammals, are oriented to belong. The lineage of the psychotherapist is majorly influenced by the priest and the doctor.[5] Their performances and shadows are part of our inheritance.

The Shadows and Performances are not for every person in the field; it's probably a large portion, but not everyone. This chapter is not speaking to the workers that are clearly doing this work for a paycheck to survive; they have less incentive to hide their shadow from themselves. This also is not for the people who consciously look to use the shadow of these professions for personal power. This is for us, who judge those people for not "caring enough." This is for us, myself included, who believe we are doing good work and serving "selflessly." We are the ones who often have had to hide our secret needs and desires that bring us to this performance, even from ourselves.

Let us begin with the priest. Their role was to protect society from itself. Because of the evolution of Christian doctrine, people were naturally bad, and their lives should have been dedicated to becoming good. The priest's role was to protect the purity of their doctrine and to help individuals overcome their natural badness. The priest was still probably closer to what we see as a shaman today than to a Catholic priest of today. They could hold rituals and actually work on behalf of God. To hold onto this powerful position, the priest could not express doubt. Which led to what Guggenbühl-Craig calls the shadow of the false prophet.[6] The priests had to perform their doubtlessness. The false prophet shadow side could account for the historical and ongoing abuse or hypocrisy we continue to uncover about those who hold "spiritual power." The priest must perform complete faith without any doubt that they are a good person as well, and they do this by always appearing to follow the doctrine. This means that any desire, thought or impulse that negates or threatens their performance must be cast away through suppression or active hiding.

This suppression or hiding is not limited to them but encouraged in the people going to the priest for help as well. When interacting with the priest, individuals were pressured to put aside their own doubt, brought on by intuition, in exchange for faith in the sureness of the priest. Since the parishioners were so disembodied, it made it easy for them to ignore their own limbic doubts in favor of the false prophet. The priest became not only a place to ensure they were on the right path leading away from eternal damnation but also to learn what of themselves they should suppress. What they did not know then was that they were creating a private life and inner world, which would lead to our compulsion towards finding authenticity, healing feelings of innate unworthiness and a fear of an inner monster.

The doctor, on the other hand, was more removed from the spiritual foundations of their role; however, they were (are) still seen as a "wise man" rather than the punitive authority figure they are. The doctor is "feared, respected, hated and admired, he seems at times an almost godlike redeemer."[6] The doctors of early hospitals were extensions of the judiciary of government.[2] Unlike their priest ancestors, instead of seeing all people as bad and helping make them good, they believed something was wrong with some people that made them lazy or ignorant, and with enough work, effort, training and discipline, the ailment could be healed. Once rehabilitated, these ill people could then rejoin the "healthy and modern" society. So, if these people were ill, then the doctors could not be seen as ill themselves. This creates the shadow of the charlatan.[6] This performance must include demonstrating the health they are prescribing to the individuals coming to them or demonstrating that they believe it.[6] This means when someone comes to this helper, there is a performance of the doctor that must showcase that not only are these norms achievable, but that they themselves have achieved them.

This again means desires, thoughts and impulses that are "unhealthy" must be suppressed or actively hidden. When a doctor works without awareness of the performance or shadow, "the doctor is no longer able to see his own wounds, his own potential for illness; he sees sickness only in the other. He objectifies illness, distances himself from his own weakness, elevates himself and degrades the patient."[6]

It would be simple and easy to call this all the past, but I hope by now you get that nothing is that simple; these shadows and performances still exist today. Doctors still hide behind their intellect, using it as a defense mechanism from being present. Theory becomes a mechanism to hide behind and protect their superiority.[7] Theory allows the doctor to be unmoved by the client's suffering and see it as neutral.[5] In actuality, the distance between the professional and the patient has become greater as technology advances and doctors can rely on technology to further themselves from the ill.[8]

Notice that both performances of these professions must be experts, which is an ideal trait in this culture. They cannot appear unsure, which is very unattractive to voluntary groups. Remember that performing competence and confidence keeps shame away, and feeling shame is unacceptable here. The doctor and the professions following, including psychotherapists, use the newest part of the brain, the neocortical brain, abandoning the limbic that has the road map for the disconnection we are trying to treat. This explains why, in the modern day, so many people are looking to "alternative medicines" or new-age spirituality, and there is a growing abandonment of the authority of medicine.[8] People are seeing the shadow side, that these authority figures actually don't have the answers and that if they do not know, they will never admit it. Scarily, people are not seeing the psychotherapist in this bucket, especially since the psychotherapist has strived for the validation of being in this bucket. It makes sense why people have been going to the jungle for psychedelics for "indigenous healing." However, we must remember that the psychedelic industry, as it is rolling out in the US, is in the lineage of medicine, not of indigenous practice. American psychedelic-assisted psychotherapy is aligned with the intellect, not our limbic knowing. And we must wonder who gets the stamp of approval as "indigenous" for Western consumption.

As I mentioned earlier, these shadows are not designated to certain people, but part of the professions themselves, yet are more intensively seen (or unseen) in those who deeply align with the good nature of the work they are doing. Yes, that means the more "good" you think you are doing, probably the more seeped in shadow you are. I argue that these shadows are distinctly Western and that they come from a culture that evolved to be more comfortable with the performance of power rather than the vulnerability of intuition. The more we align with the performance, the greater the dispositionalism we implore to protect the image. That means we go on to ignore where there are contradictions in ourselves in the role of helper, or in the systems we are within, and even the people we are claiming to help. The more we align with the fundamental attribution error, the more we rely on our "good" work to prove we are generally "good" people.

Finally, the last two ancestral lineages of the psychotherapist, the police and charity/case worker have their own shadows. Although I will not be extensively going into these, there are plenty of people who do. I will highlight two glaring enactments of modern shadow parts of these professions. One is that police performance is to surveil, report and detain people who are a harm to society, and yet a federal questionnaire of police officers found that upwards of 40 percent of police polled *self-reported* being physically violent with their spouses in the previous six months.[9] That was 40 percent who self-reported; can you imagine how many actually are physically violent with their spouses? Or the shadow of charity/case workers who perform that they believe everyone deserves the right to live a good life, and yet a study of the 1970s and 80s on burnout showed that after time, they had less empathy and felt more numb, even expressed bitterness, resentment and *even hate towards their clients.*[10] I know, a good anti-oppressive therapist hates being compared to the police, but we are trained towards similar goals. Which is why it disturbs me when I hear the response to police brutality is not to defund and abolish it; it's to add social workers to their roster. *Rolls eyes.*

All of these performances occur because there cannot be any honesty about the role and purpose of the helper. Any honesty would interrupt the collective cognitive dissonance needed to sustain the status quo. In the West, with our lack of kinship and storytelling elders, socially we are not looking at the historical legacy of these professions. If I were told that the role of the helper was to gaslight people into feeling they are falling short of a fictional standard of normal that was created to make people profitable for the government, I might not have gone to social work school.

Feel Into It

Well? How does it make you feel to be compared to the police?

Practice to Intervention

I had a professor in grad school who taught a class on trauma, and she created many opportunities to switch from using our neocortex to feeling into our limbic system. And that included encouraging us to have feelings in class. The class often included a circle of crying students; I thought it was a waste of time. Although there was a setting issue (being in grad school with a bunch of white women), I also could not allow myself to be heartbroken about the impossibility of our work at the time because my performance and self-worth were wrapped up in feeling good and valuable by being a helper. And now my heartbrokenness leads my work.

Can you see how the feeling that came up in response to being compared to the police is familiar to you? Can you begin to imagine what that feeling has to teach you about some shadow work you may have waiting?

Because the priest, the doctor, the police, the charity/case worker and the psychotherapist utilize the neocortex, they exploit the limbic system that is oriented towards depending on others; we over-promise and under-deliver.

The Professional Helper

But professions are not people. You may be asking, "Why do these shadows of professionals also speak to the shadow of the people practicing them?" Because these shadows also match our shadows. In the West, mature adulting is achieved when you have created a life that matches the performance you want to have. What we aren't consciously admitting to is that the life we want to live must also protect our shadow.

And because I love what I do, I must still say it takes a special kind of person, in a world of dissonance, to choose to witness and confront people's truths. In some ways, the helpers are people who have the grandiosity needed to believe they can change things. And as we saw in Chapter 4, to have this type of grandiosity, you need to shove some other things away.

When the helper was a young person, they probably found being a helper to be their strong suit. Strong suits are not only characteristics that are acceptable in this culture; they are ones that are admirable; they earn praise and value. There becomes an addiction to receiving this admiration. Like, "Gosh, I could never do what you do," or "Wow, we need more people like you in the world" or "Thank you, I couldn't have done this without you." We keep striving to feel the temporary rush of endorphins we receive with those sentiments, but they never satisfy.[5] I am not saying we should not let those comments sink in and nourish us, but we must also be aware when we are chasing them and they are not nourishing us. And without awareness of this, we will seek it out and protect it with little regard for what we may give up. In some ways, what was a strong suit becomes a "psychological failure"[6] because it originated as a tenderness towards the suffering of others and is now used to gain and maintain personal power. It actually evolves to push away tenderness and hide shame.

Shame in communal cultures draws people in towards each other. In this society, shame causes individuals to become withdrawn and less curious.[1] Remember that to hide shame, we must appear competent. This competence must suggest we are already knowledgeable, which decreases our curiosity and openness to being receptive to new or conflicting information or tolerate being caught as wrong. This feels antithetical to being a therapist. However, as people who are trained to ask a lot of questions, I am honestly constantly disappointed by the amount of clinicians I encounter who are quite nice but narrow-sighted and cannot tolerate conflicting information. They appear offended and uninterested in being curious or differing perspectives. They tend to stay in their like-minded voluntary organizations where they can remain that way. I cannot hide behind putting it off only on other therapists. I have been that therapist and still can be now. Especially when I am overwhelmed, I become that therapist again because the initial energy it takes to keep my walls up is less than the energy it takes to stay open.

Feel Into It

Is this at all familiar to you, in yourself? How do you know when you are walled up and when you are open? What happens in your body that signals this to you? Check in front of your chest, behind your back, the tilt of your hips, the energy in your legs.

The issue with building our walls or wearing a disguise is that the person we were intended to serve pays the price. We become less curious about the person in front of us and more concerned with the maintenance of our disguise of competence. When our energy is going towards maintaining the disguise, we fall into the trap of using our clients to fulfill our needs. Devon Price offers their experience for our learning when they share, "Browbeaten . . . into hiding every vulnerability and need and left me obsessed with proving my worth to other people . . . Whenever I felt lonely or sad, I would try to boost my mood by helping somebody else."[10]

I know I have found myself leaving a session "high" because so much "good work" happened, and I felt integral in the process. Or felt deflated after a session where I felt useless. This impacts our work and the people we serve. Only the professional and the one being served know what happens in the hour they spend together. In some ways, this places the practitioner in the tower of their own panopticon. The person in the down-power position (client, patient) must perform for their doctor, and with our curiosity down, we will take our client's improvement as the boost we need rather than having curiosity about it. Since the practitioner themselves are still using their performance and shadow to get what they want, there is an unrealized belief that the performance is as good as having the longing met. So, the practitioner may not push against the client's performance and accept it as signs of improvement. The patient can satisfy the practitioner's desire to be seen as wise and kind by giving information that will align with what the professional expects.[7] This acceptance of performance and lack of curiosity often leaves the client to take responsibility not only for the healing of their pain but for the social and cultural dysfunction that caused their pain and that of their professional "helper."

Remember Kris from Chapter 2? Let me help jog our memory. They were a fictional character in an image used in a study. In the image, they are standing in front of a group. The study showed Japanese participants looked at the whole group to determine how Kris felt, while Americans only looked at Kris, ignoring the others. Ok, so it is basically like saying Kris is happy because they are smiling even though everyone else in the background is frowning and seems to be throwing eye daggers at Kris. The amount of energy it takes to keep up performances makes us lack curiosity about the relationship between things, allowing us to ignore what would complicate the situation. We abandon nuance in exchange for protecting our point of view or ego.

And if we clinicians are invested in protecting our egos, then our clients who are primed not to trust their own instincts, like we all are in this culture, are left to our mercy. Due to this power difference, the professional cannot be held accountable by the person they serve; they do not need to accept or integrate feedback given.[11] In fact, those clients who reject this automatic trust and do not abandon themselves are seen as resistant. At that point, the professional can scold the person they are serving rather than take in feedback about what is happening in the relational field. In these types of dynamics, the practitioner is so fragile they cannot take any conflictual information, so they cannot be truly present or in limbic resonance with their client.[11]

This lack of openness and avoidance of accountability puts clients in a double bind where they came in to get help but must lie to the helper. This reminds me of the many times in a doctor's office, they ask about something and I have a conflict in my mind of what I want to respond with because, although they are saying, "You can tell me anything," I know they will judge me and speak as though I deserve my ailment. This creates that bind where I want to be honest, but I expect the practitioner will judge me so I do not say everything (lying by omission), and then I feel guilty for being dishonest and the doctor gets to walk away, superiority intact. Being in a downpower position, a client, patient, person you serve or myself actually puts us in the position to not have our needs met.[1] That is part of the expectation of downpower, that their needs can be overlooked for the up-power person.

Practice to Intervention

Just me? Do you know what I am talking about? What happens in you when you must consider whether you can tell the truth or not to someone you are supposed to be honest with? Can you feel it now?
  Or
  Do you know that feeling when you feel someone is telling you what they think you want to hear but can't be sure? What do you take it to mean? What impulses arise in response?

Shadow Protectors

The industry of psychotherapy is created to make good people out of a bad culture. In the United States, "self-help technologies" arose to respond to the isolation individuals experienced during the Industrial Revolution and after the trauma of civil war. These technologies "taught Americans to reframe the adversity of the era as an internal problem with individual-level solutions."[12] Psychoanalysis came along and picked up the self-help torch and enhanced the skill set of adapting to the oppressive norms of the culture. Then came behaviorism that focused on changing the response a person has to their context and finally, humanism that solidified that internally is where all our focus should go.

These perspectives of therapy rely on a set of theories. I call those our shadow protectors. They help us feel competent and knowledgeable. Some of the dominant theories that sustain the field of psychology and social services were and still are in service of protecting power and the status quo. They concretize the culture as normal, the client as deviant, and the therapist as the remedy. Even models that are looking to move away from oppressive methods often see these as fundamental to human behavior and do not question their validity.

So, of course, I question them. I am going to critique some of our favorite theories that undergird development in the West. Although they are made up, they are true for people conditioned in them. There is value in learning these theories because they shape our world. I only ask that we hold them gingerly as the fragile things they are. I will name specific theorists in the next section, not to blame them since they were simply the ones recognized for capturing the cultural consciousness of their time.

Let's talk a bit about social Darwinism, again. Darwinism, and especially social Darwinism, continues to be used as a theory to protect hierarchy and create the illusion of there being a natural way of being. This way of being justifies much violence in our culture and exporting it throughout the world. Natural often is meant as "self-occurring" or autopoietic. However, "critters do not precede their relatings," Donna Haraway reminds us.[13] Even within seemingly single-celled microorganisms, like the M. paradoxa, under advanced microscopes, five distinct beings exist within it. And these beings, without the right conditions and each other, cannot be the single-celled organism.

Our interpretation of evolution and Darwinism is wrong. We, and all beings, are actually sympoietic, meaning these systems are needed for the existence of other beings and are actually not separate.[13] Sympoietic is "making with" or "becoming with." Most things that exist now have not been naturally selected; they have been artificially selected. We have given value to some beings and created the conditions for their sustainability while destroying the conditions for beings we consider disposable that begin to decline in existence. Our preference for the autopoietic idea of evolution is part of our cognitive dissonance. It allows us to pretend there are some natural and uncontrollable forces at play, which relieves us of any responsibility of what lives, what dies, what suffers, what goes extinct. Genetics are not solo in their development and do not explain why people are or do what they do. Genetics are so slow. Cultural evolution is more informative of who exists and survives than biology. Epigenetics is the new Darwinism, as in it is misused as a predisposition that will explain everything. Yes, you can have genetic markers from an earlier generation, imprints on the genes, but allostatic load, the measurement of stress on the body, influences the body in that it can instigate the imprints to activate or not. It is actually a way to adapt without permanency.[5] So epigenetics is not actually about genes changing; it is about the context that impacts the readiness of a gene to activate.

"To the extent that we cling to genetic fundamentalism to avoid the discomforts of personal responsibility or societal reckoning, we radically- and unnecessarily-disempower ourselves from dealing either actively or proactively with suffering of all kinds."[5] As I have said a few times already, although genes matter, social conditioning, caregiving and environmental influences can override genetics. This resignation to genetics often leaves clients and us to take the simplest out, which is to say something is genetic and therefore unable to be different, when, in fact, it most likely is cultural and not a curse of genes.

Then there is Freud, whose "assumptions have endured for so many years that they are mistaken for fact."[8] His theories lacked any importance given to social context and sadly internalized the consciousness that was of the time. The inner private world that the priests were trying to extinguish centuries earlier returns as the devil's playground and a threat to society. The only remedy is confession, humiliation and then to be returned to being a secret. This evil, the "death instinct" that lurked inside looked to destroy ourselves and others by obstructing the ability to be "normal" and could spring up at any time.[1]

He made all types of rules that he himself did not follow; for all of his obsession with transference and being a blank slate, he analyzed his friends, his daughter and had many dual relationships. Freud clearly used this to try to get his feeling of belonging met. He protected his fragile power by rewarding clients who "remembered" latent sexual desire and called primitive or underdeveloped those who denied such memory or inclinations.[8] And if this latent evil never appears, then that only shows the power of repression in the client and their lack of work. Essentially a client who fails to prove his theory still proves it. Again, that double bind. In many ways, this is Freud training people to create this inner world that is a secret even to themselves. This does, in fact, change the emotional landscape of Westerners and make us psychologically and emotionally peculiar to the global majority. What was actually being suppressed is our connective nature, to be replaced by an individual "internal world." Freud also solidified the place of the psychoanalyst to contain an omnipotent and "quasi-divine" posture.[2] And that power still exists and impacts lives, the power to declare someone as "abnormal" or "unhealthy."

And then there is Abraham Maslow and his hierarchy of needs. It is still seen as the model on how to prioritize needs and decide who deserves care. If you were to do a quick Google search of the theory right now, you would find many sites repeating the belief that to get to self-actualization, which is "the goal of life," we must meet the lower-ranking needs and move up the chain. This is another internalization of the belief that the population is made up of a mass of indistinguishable people and only a few, through hard work and standing out in the crowd, can have a successful life.[14]

But let's put this in perspective. Maslow was a researcher of motivation, basically "what will get people to do things." His whole work was how to get people motivated to conform to social norms. He also utilized Western entitlement and individualism to re-work indigenous wisdom. He was inspired to create his model from his time with Blood First Nations indigenous peoples.[15] Indigenous scholars are clear that Maslow did not accurately depict the framework of needs he appropriated from Blood First Nations.

They differ in three major ways. First, he made it about an individual life, whereas for the Blood First Nations, these were multi-generational centers of life and not about individual self-actualization. The second major divergence made was that he made them hierarchical when the framework would be better presented in concentric circles. Lastly, unlike the Indigenous framework, Maslow's original hierarchy did not include spirituality. Maslow later revised the hierarchy, adding above Self-Actualization, Transcendence.[16] Transcendence is where people begin looking outside of themselves and their egos and begin looking to help others. This comes after self-actualization, which includes some sort of financial wealth as well. Transcendence is where we begin thinking about other beings and "sharing the wealth."

"Individuation is not something which can be acquired and then securely owned . . . it is symbolically described in such images as 'the journey to the golden city.'"[6] This journey is always happening as long as arrival to perfection has not been acquired, which means individuation requires never-ending work and effort, which of course is perfect for the state. Again, this model is an internalization of an elitist aesthetic of a good life, which already permeated collective consciousness. Mesquita and Henrich give examples and make sure to point out how pointless accruing wealth is in other cultures. In collectivist cultures, people share what they have. In some, it does not even make sense to strive for personal wealth since it will always be shared with their kin, so it's lost as soon as it's gained. In these cultures, transcendence is basic, not the highest level of human development.

Let's move on to Pavlov and his dogs. Pavlov's more famous finding was that if you reward something, it is more likely to reinforce the behavior, wiring it into habit. He proved this by holding a bunch of dogs hostage in his basement. This is another exercise on training beings to perform desired behaviors and norms. His less popular finding was an accident; those same dogs were trapped in cages when there was a flood in his basement and most of them stopped responding to stimuli altogether while others became hyper-vigilant towards all stimuli.[17] So all of that positive reinforcement and negative reinforcement went down the drain (pun intended) when there was an actual trauma to these dogs. So, conditioning these dogs into norms did not actually change their nature; it just trained them away from their own rhythms and instincts. Pavlov did note after this that what did change was the dogs had drastically low to no curiosity about their environment after trauma. After having their ability to respond authentically stripped away by being in cages, they lost all curiosity. We find again that suppression dampens curiosity.

I feel we do not spend enough time speaking about this part, that these dogs were captive. These dogs were not home; they were not where they had power; they were made dependent on Pavlov. This only proves if you exercise power over another being, they will conform to survive. This is an exercise in power. What Pavlov actually proved was that if you force a being to be completely reliant on you, they will do as you train them to do so they can get their needs met. These dogs were made reliant via moving them in an unnatural setting (dislocation), therefore restraining them from being able to follow their instincts toward getting their needs met (stripping of ritual, rites and norms) and then attaching their survival needs to their ability to perform (suppression). Colonization 101. It is also how research is generally done in hyper-controlled, isolated contexts where we put animals through a basic level of torture/colonization and then prove it is human nature. This is done in research, and research is done in therapeutic settings.

We also know this is not human nature. Remember that game mentioned in Chapter 3? If you were to punish or negatively reinforce players of the game that were not Westerners, they would not cooperate; they would instead retaliate. They would actually be more likely to fight back or to give out their own punishments. While Western players were more likely to cooperate after receiving punishment. And so there's something inherently incorrect about our cultural assimilation of Pavlov's original theory into a general understanding of human nature. Coming out of our cultural evolution that uplifts obedience and discipline, it is true, but it is not natural.

Practice to Intervention

What are the questions you have now? What has been confirmed? What do you suspect you will be grappling with? Talk it out with your group.

The Professional Landscape

How are these theories so widely accepted and unquestioned? Because they validate our cultural values, and our institutions have no incentive to reconsider. The psychological industry was erected out of elites wanting to tame and control the population. We are "aiming to make us more functional in dysfunctional systems, rather than awakening investigation so we can challenge the system itself."[11] Thanissara is speaking of Western Buddhism in this quote, but I feel it can be used in the overlapping Industrial Complexes we work in Medical, Non-Profit, Prison, etc. Not being able to "rise above" our conditions is seen as an issue of weakness and laziness, but not about the conditions we are asking people to "rise above."

These helping groups became organizations following the Civil War; they offered charity to "those seen to be 'deserving' of assistance, such as widows and children. These charities focused on individual poverty rather than poverty on the systemic level."[18] This charity model of helping whom the state finds deserving becomes the non-profit sector. Becoming organizations consumed with accomplishing their short-term goals that prove their necessity rather than getting to the root of the issue.

The structures we work in are the watered-down institutional rip-offs of kinship work. They make the client-practitioner relational field lack honesty and vulnerability. In our professions, sustaining caseloads is a part of guaranteeing our survival.[19] The number of clients a professional has to see is increasing; we are asked to do more with less and the illusion of safety nets that once existed is no longer. Due to cultural evolution that informs that everything is possible through hard work and discipline, helping professionals are seen as a kind gesture. Increasingly, the financial cost of care is being prioritized in determining the quality of care that can be offered or that is deserved.[20] I have worked for more than one organization where the people who dictated how I should work had no idea about what my actual job was but had a lot of theories and statistics on how I could do it better. By better, they always meant more efficient and with less resources.

During and since the Industrial Revolution, these foundations, non-profits and partial public entities have tackled the difficult work of protecting the wealthy and the oppressive systems that make them possible. Charity, non-profits and foundations are the elite's transcendence. After reaching "self-actualization," they can start "caring" for others. Since these organizations are a part of these wealthy people's personal journey, the organizations take cues from the wealthy on how to use their money, time and personnel. These are the training containers for students in the psychotherapeutic field and often are the first places we work. Under close surveillance and supervision, psychotherapists learn the fundamentals of running a practice. Many of these fundamentals were inherited from the early hospital.

Fundamental number 1: Build rapport, but rapport often translates to "make sure they trust you to be their authority." We are taught how to impart the image of sageness to maintain this domination. How to nod and gesture. Even if not explicitly told, we are modeled how to speak as though we know something the client does not know about themselves.[6] We are expected to "deliver insight."[8] This assures that our clients see us as an authority figure and a little "all-knowing."

Fundamental number 2: Stay separate. In our disgust at interconnectedness, we will help our clients to become more independent and pathologize dependence.[8] It is worthy of investigation if our clients or ourselves begin to actually care for each other. In a world run by power shadow, I agree that dual relationships should be entered with much support and cautiously, not because they are bad, but because, in a culture like ours, it's a recipe for abuse. Yet, dual relationships are how accountability can happen. When we ignore the relational field, which we do in our practice settings, we are enabling disconnection, colluding with the beliefs that healthy relationships are detached, transactional and have intrinsic power dynamics that must be protected.

Third fundamental: Take orderly notes. It was a sign of a good doctor in the early hospital as it transitioned into a science of experts to have records that helped locate individuals.[2] "But documentation does not help one perceive. At best it only analyzes the perception."[21] These records, which at once are used to remember clients, become data points for future use. Think of the future, like data analysis or subpoena; think surveillance. This makes individuals banks of knowledge to extract from in order to create/maintain wealth and sustain power. This is the same colonized model that has been used by Westerners around the world in their pursuit of infinite wealth and power. We turn people and societies "into objects we would sooner study than learn from."[22]

The records also included examination. Think about how many questions we ask in an intake that are unnecessary to their treatment or their particular desires but need to be collected.[3]

Which leads us to Fundamental 4: Examination or evaluation is a must. It is where the individual is objectified, categorized and made into cases of illness or "otherness." This is how the helpee knows they need you. Once you have diagnosed their problem(s), you must be generous and willing to help. Evaluations make sense because of healthism. Because the helpee has come in contact with the medical-industrial complex, we must assess all of their health. "Healthism is the belief that health is a moral imperative and individual responsibility."[23] Which means they may come in for one thing, but we must judge them on their health in other areas as well. The thing with healthism is that it is based on the professional's perception of health, not on the client's experience.

Fundamental number 5: There is always more that can be done. The effectiveness of the treatment is based on the client's ability and "capacity" to work. And that work is always to make them a good, healthy and normal member of society.

Us Western practitioners of the helping profession cannot be present with what is; we are always future-focused.[6] All of these contribute to a lack of authentic relating in our current psychological field and alignment with oppressive forces. No, these are not mad scientists scheming in the lab, nor are they perverse vigilante social experimenters running fantasies in their basements. Although there are examples of practitioners who have fully embraced their shadow, the scary stuff is not dramatic or heroic; they are subtle and accepted as common sense practice, like the fundamentals listed above.

The Helpee

Who is this scary stuff happening to? Well, all of us, through social conditioning done at home, school, media and our general limbic disconnect. It also happens in the therapeutic relationship. Who we help are those who are not able or not willing to comply with social norms. And this profession has created life work out of wrangling what we find ugly and keeping them occupied with becoming desirable so they do not disturb the status quo. When I use ugly here, I mean it in the way Da'Shaun L. Harrison uses it. "Ugly is political. It is the determiner for who does and does not work, who does and does not receive love, who does and does not die, who does and is not eat, who is and is not housed."[24] Although they are referring to the literal traits society finds physically repulsive, I mean who we cognitively find repulsive, too; who we must hide to keep our "perfect cities" and who we must find repulsive to protect our own ugliness. And they know they are repulsive. Therapy is like a secret agreement that we will make you pretty enough.

Early hospital days, the helpee was the madman. Today, we would use words like crazy, psychotic, mentally unstable, problematic, disruptive, etc. The madman "must feel morally responsible for everything within him that may disturb morality and society, and must hold no one but himself responsible for the punishment he receives."[2] We are the punishment; we are the punishers. How often, in response to something disapproving, people suggest that someone "see a therapist?" Therapy is where you get corrected (see punished).

At one point in history, the madman was possessed or just ignorant; in the height of the hospital, the madman became someone who was secretly aware of their madness and must be shown to themselves to correct themselves. This approach to the madman has not gone away, it still is the perspective we take of the helpee. This is the belief that our work is to make people confront themselves. That if they really saw themselves, they wouldn't like what they saw, and they'd do something different.

The helpee is the person who bears the responsibility for failing to be normal, healthy or good. And they are coming to us to work harder at correcting this cosmic mistake. Some people fail themselves, they go to the therapist; some people fail the "bourgeois," they go to prison.[2] For these people, they become a criminal. But many people we call criminals were criminals before they committed the crime because of the ways they were ugly. In other words, being poor makes you a criminal before you commit a crime, being Black, Indigenous or other POC makes you a criminal before you commit a crime; being Trans, Genderfluid or Queer makes you a criminal before you commit a crime. This is the delinquent. And the non-profit complex makes itself the savior that keeps you from committing the crime you have already been blamed for. The creation of the delinquent came out of hospitals, and it was basically saying that the life the person lives, or had to live, made them a criminal before they committed the crime.

One example is the Carnegie and Rockefeller Foundations' hired eugenicist (see MIC scientist) to study who they perceived as delinquents. "This science was then used to prove that someone's genetic makeup was the root cause of poverty: having a predilection to criminality, substance use, or a tendency toward homosexuality, to name a few."[25] Another example is to eliminate homosexuality, psychedelic clinical research (again see MIC science) has attempted to erase the deviant from themselves by using psychedelics in conversion therapy in recent history.[26] These are examples of acceptable scientific pursuits that were used to prove that delinquents caused their suffering, therefore, they needed to be saved from themselves.

How many non-profits are geared around the purpose of keeping young black, brown and poor kids "off of the streets?" What they are inadvertently admitting is that they believe these children are already criminals, and it is a matter of keeping them out of the right place, right time, to prevent them from committing the crime. It is like a race "to get them before the street does." Where the prize is getting to claim ownership of their reformation. There is no curiosity around, "How can we put a whole neighborhood into the category of criminal, a whole race, a whole class of people?"

"Programs are proposed and implemented that penalize black women and their children for the crime of being poor."[27] Survival is criminalized. The crime that us criminals have committed is taking our lives so seriously that we are willing to do what it takes to survive.[28] How can we devote so much energy towards policy or reform without trying to understand the cultural belief that whole groups of people deserve hardship? I have been told many times and in many ways that those questions are out of our scope or are distracting the purpose.

Sadly, our commitment to staying in our "purpose" contributes to the destruction of these people who often have lessons for us about the kinship this culture is starving for.

The eugenic science affirmed the cultural beliefs to blame the helpee "for their conditions based on genetics as opposed to structural violence."[25] This science is what is informing our fields. If these systems were truly about change, they would take their cue from the people they claim they want to help. Black, Brown, Indigenous, Queer people have rallied around the safety and needs of their communities as long as these systems existed and worked to protect each other from them. These practices were part of creating belonging, but today would be a strategy under the umbrella of Liberatory Harm Reduction.

> Liberatory Harm Reduction came through the Black Panthers' creation of free breakfast programs to feed and nourish a revolution, and through the Young Lords' occupation of Lincoln Hospital in the Bronx to demand- and ultimately operate- community-run, accessible drug treatment programs.[28]

Immigrants, as long as forever, had lessons on how to keep each other safe and well. These groups were kin-based. But rather than being seen as a blueprint, they were seen as threats; they were targeted, disconnected and eliminated. What was stolen from them were state-sanctioned, watered-down individualist versions of community. Our organizations do not take their cue from these communities because of this notion of epistemic justice. Epistemic justice is the wrong done to people that invalidates their ability to be authorities of their own experiences or trusted as knowers of their needs and the solutions to their needs.[23]

The helpees are also people who fall out of spiritual allowance. "For the nineteenth century, the initial model of madness would be to believe oneself to be god, while for the preceding centuries it had been to deny god."[2] Prior to that and still around the world, "people with visions may become prophets or shamans,"[5] but here and now, they are only hallucinating. There are some exceptions in the psychedelic-assisted psychotherapy world. However, since the medical industrial complex is "non-spiritual," there are tensions about what to do with spiritual visions. Let us not forget that visions are impacted by culture. In the early hospitals, when people started having visions of scary demons or an angry god, the hospitals took down spiritual images, and it greatly improved the treatment outcomes of their captives.[2] Which was how the hospital and medical industry began shedding their spiritual beginnings. With that understanding, those who plan to do work in the Psychedelic assisted therapy field must keep in mind visions are still impacted by context, culture and history. Our visions in the West go through a Western interpretation system. Those visions are not exempt from socialization. I hear and see a lot of visuals that are still very self-centered, grandiose and towards our own happiness and purpose. Not to say they aren't valuable, but here, too, we must hold the tension. Helpees can also be people who are pathologized for believing in something that the culture doesn't uplift as normal or possible.

If the helpees are not in an undervalued identity group that is criminalized for existing, they are coming to us because the goodness, healthiness or normalness they seek is elusive, and, due to entitlement, it shouldn't be that way for them. They want to find the magical switch inside of themselves that will help them to become a better person, a person who deserves happiness.

If the helpee has had an incident in their life that they believe has interrupted their happiness, they may come to counseling. Usually, we would call this trauma. As I shared in Chapter 1, we live in a sociopathic society. If you live in a sociopathic society, then you are traumatized. Bessel van der Kolk writes,

> [B]eing traumatized means continuing to organize your life as if the trauma were still going on – unchanged and immutable – as every encounter or event is contaminated by the past . . . The survivors energy now becomes focused on suppressing inner chaos.[17]

There are "big T" traumas where there is a clear event with a before and after, but what about the rest of us? When the before is preverbal? When the event is being disembodied as early as sleep training? We are a culture consumed with "suppressing inner chaos." The issue of the profession is that we prioritize trauma that interrupts our functionality. We do this because our culture sees a happy, easy and productive life as our right, as the "natural course of things," and if something "interrupts" the course, it is trauma. This ignores sympoiesis that we become with each other. That life is made up of things, people, places and even incidents becoming together. Life is not meant to be comfortable or happy; it just is. We do not give the label or attention to the trauma of limbic disconnection that is pervasive because it keeps us searching, looking and working for that elusive happy life that we can earn. That trauma is actually functional. That same disconnection, however, brings about the big T traumas that cause more pain and more suffering. Shira Hassan appeals that "we need to start considering trauma as a macro concept thinking through how living in the constant reality or repeated and daily trauma impacts people on an individual level."[28]

Practice to Intervention

We are primed to make ourselves useful and productive. Noticing macro on an individual can sound like "I want to make a difference" or "What is my purpose?"

By seeing these questions as cultural, we interrupt our professional training to focus "on an individual's experience instead of structures of violence in which we live."[25] This allows space to have feelings about the macro trauma. Not allowing it to remain invisible or to seem normal.

Spend some time jotting down some issues the people you serve are working with; how are they connected to macro trauma?

So, interesting tidbit, I am really into cults; I find them to be such honest stories about our social conditioning. Although they are often seen as predatorial, they are responding to three major Western conditionings. The first is not a conditioning but actual human orientation towards being connected, being accepted and a sense of belonging. The second one is the conditioning towards a calling; for an individual life to mean more than one life, that it must leave a legacy of some sort or be worth more than one lifetime. Like wanting to matter or do something good with their life. Finally, each individual is a part of this bigger movement or body that wants to be a force of good in the world. That their efforts together will be worth more than their efforts alone. They often win over members by having a doctrine that states if you work on yourself in some form or another, have discipline, live a good and healthy life as defined by (insert cult leader name), you can either save the world or be spared when the world ends. In many ways, I see psychotherapists as recruits for this big societal cult.

We push very similar beliefs that by each individual being better, we can save our planet. But as we read in Chapter 2, these ideals were created so societies could scale up and maintain order and control. These ideals are what keep us isolated, disconnected from our bodies, our spirits, land and other beings. These ideals keep us competing, making us restless and grandiose yet always dissatisfied. In many ways, we, like cult recruiters, make promises that if they just keep at it, they will make it to the next level or some promised land, one that we haven't reached yet, but promise will happen.

Psychotherapy

Psychotherapy is where we train people to be normal, healthy and good. Like many cult recruiters, it often is not because of malice or wishing harm on someone, it is because we believe the message, too, or are looking to protect ourselves.

Instead of being honest that the same oppression that is torturing and traumatizing our clients we are suffering from as well, we either idolize clients, being in awe of their resilience or feeling their pain "was for a reason." The other side is that we judge them as unwilling to "get it together" and deserving of their hardship. If you work for a non-profit, you are either touting them around at your fundraiser or talking shit about them in the staff lounge. The ones we like and are in "awe" of, we work harder to help them find a job or go back to school because we think they deserve another chance to be a productive member of society again. In private practice, we might see whether a client is succeeding or not as a result of our work and effort or their lack of work or effort.

Therapy in this society is committed to ignoring this traumatic society and "reforming people" to return to this traumatic society. Still traumatized but better equipped to cope or more empowered to do their share of the traumatizing themselves.

If we have not learned to be disillusioned, we will carelessly indoctrinate people into the cult of the West. We can follow the profession's example and use our authority to get them back in good favor with a toxic culture, or we can use our position to give their authority back to them. Reminding them that their authority is internal and giving them permission to take it away from society and take it away from us as well.

Abandoning the Profession

Is there another way to be? Yes, but is the cost high? Definitely. First,

> we must question our role as agents of the state when being asked to control or surveil bodies, families, and communities under the guise of "safety" or "for the public good or well-being," when it oftentimes can lead to irrevocable harm.[25]

We must admit that "our reliance on policing to keep 'us' 'safe' results in the extension of policing behaviors in our everyday lives and culture."[25] These ways of being go on to make up organizations and industries that are sustained by policing. Then,

> we have to disrupt them. And not disrupt them by trying to figure out how to be on their boards and trying to figure out how to do their diversity committees; we have to disrupt them by saying "I am out." I'm not going to participate in this and letting them know why.[19]

The "them," the "they," I wish I could say, are specific organizations, but I think for us, it's the profession itself.

Now, I know we all cannot quit our jobs, let our licenses lapse and live off-grid (big dreams of mine). But what is your movement in that direction? What if we abandoned the role of the helper? What if we raged against this profession? What if we used our hearts that want to help, that want to give and receive care and detached them from the helping professions? What if we disconnected our natural need for belonging from the labor we do for survival?

I invite us, you reading and myself, to consider what it would be like if we were to split apart our needs from the work we do for survival. If we stopped promising liberation through confessing and instead liberation through not performing. There is a difference. Confessing, as we have seen, has a moral value that through confession there is a route to make someone good again; admitting to their wrongdoings and wrong thoughts is a way to purify. Confession is the penance for not being normal, healthy or good; it can be redemptive. By purging all of the life experiences and traumas that have shaped them, they will be able to finally be normal, live a happy and healthy life.

However, an invitation not to perform means the clinician can hold a stance of "I am not invested in you being happy, healthy or normal, I am interested in you being you right now and you feeling you right now. There isn't a better version of you before or after. You now are complete – scars, pains and all. No one is unscathed in this collective. We are sympoietic; we become with each other. Part of being is being impacted by what is around you."

The clinician can only take that stance if they know this for themselves. It is an act that comes when we have connected to our erotic power, and we give our work its erotic value back.[29] We do this by increasing our limbic capacity and attention to our own limbic system where that knowledge lives. Without this strengthening, "a therapist is fatally apt to substitute inference for resonance."[8] Without fully feeling the difference between being limbically attuned with self and simply speaking softly while making educated guesses, we will miss the possibilities to be with what is right there with us.

Let's begin by wondering how much we are missing out on. I love this question they pose in *The General Theory of Love*: "Who knows how many scientific revolutions have been missed because their potential inaugurators disregard the whimsical, the incidental, the inconvenient inside the laboratory?"[8]

Go for whimsical and inconvenient! To do this, we would need to abandon the idea that we could have successful treatment. Within the current systems in which we work, successful treatment is when we help a client conform to the illusion of societal norms. Maybe not all of the norms, but definitely the ones the clinician agrees with. To abandon the idea that we can be successful eliminates a right way of doing anything, which means we cannot be the experts; we are more like observers.

What if the clinician did not occupy the power seat? Then we would be admitting we, too, are wandering, wounded and are creating a life based on what we have available to us. This admission allows us to be accomplices to our clients as they, too, are wandering. When we make space for the invisible, the incidental, we see the collective consciousness that is with us, influencing us and lying to us. Once it is present, we can grieve. Grieve that it is the impossible task of being in this collective that leads us to wander, to feel homeless and to create something out of nothing. That nothing is actually wrong with us. This opens up the pathway to the reflection and care our limbic systems are so desperately deficient of.

Instead of focusing on corrective experiences, although we hope they occur, what if we focused on the is-ness of the matter (which we will focus on in Chapter 7). The space between the hopelessness of our conditions and the desire for something different. What if we let that unraveling of our performances and that of our clients be the place where we begin seeing our private lives are simply a clue to where there is possibility. By sifting through what was stored in the "private" pouch, we can reconnect it with all the other parts we became. As we illuminate and make visible "shadow dynamics into conscious awareness, we have to reassess what we are loyal to."[10] Empathy and compassion need a lot of energy;[9] let's stop wasting it on being normal and productive.

Let's answer this call Rev. angel Kyodo williams, Sensei, makes of us:

> Wisdom prophets who lay bare the unarmed truth of the transgenerational cultural illness of white superiority in equal measure with an unapologetic love that holds those besieged by that plague in the light of their humanity, distinguishing diseases from host, are being called forth . . . and they are gaining in number.[30]

Feel Into It

What feels possible right now? How do you know? Where in yourself does this sense of possibility rise? Check out your breath. Your heartbeat.

Citations

1. Mesquita, B. (2022). *Between us: How cultures create emotions*. W. W. Norton & Company.
2. Foucault, M., & Rabinow, P. (1984). *The Foucault reader*. Pantheon.
3. Taylor, K. (2023). *The ethics of caring: Finding right relationship with clients for profound transformative work in our professional healing relationships* (Expanded, Revised). Hanford Mead Pub.
4. Wallerstein, I. (2004). World-systems analysis. In *Duke University Press eBooks*. Duke University Press. https://doi.org/10.1215/9780822399018
5. Maté, G., MD, & Maté, D. (2022). *The myth of normal: Trauma, illness, and healing in a toxic culture*. Avery.
6. Guggenbühl-Craig, A. (1996). *Power in the helping professions* (12th ed.). Spring Publications, Inc.
7. Miller, A. (1997). *The drama of the gifted child: The search for the true self* (revised ed., 3rd ed.). Basic Books.
8. Lewis, T., Amini, F., & Lannon, R. (2001). *A general theory of love* (Reprint). Vintage.
9. Burmon, A. (2022, July 20). *Police domestic violence: Data shows 40 percent of cops abuse family*. Fatherly. www.fatherly.com/life/police-brutality-and-domestic-violence
10. Price, D., PhD. (2022). *Laziness does not exist*. Atria.
11. Thanissara. (2015). *Time to stand up: An engaged Buddhist manifesto for our earth -- The Buddha's life and message through feminine eyes (sacred activism)* (1st ed.). North Atlantic Books.
12. Brennan, B. P. (2020, August 11). *The revolution will not be psychologized: Psychedelics' potential for systemic change*. Chacruna. https://chacruna.net/the-revolution-will-not-be-psychologized-psychedelics-potential-for-systemic-change/

13. Haraway, D. J. (2016). *Staying with the trouble: Making Kin in the Chthulucene (experimental futures)* (Illustrated). Duke University Press Books.
14. Kat, S. A. (2021). *Postcolonial astrology: Reading the planets through capital, power, and labor.* North Atlantic Books.
15. Blackstock, C. (2011). The emergence of the breath of life theory. *Journal of Social Work Values and Ethics*, *8*(1).
16. Huitt, W. (2017). Hierarchy of needs. In *The SAGE encyclopedia of political behavior*. SAGE Publications. https://doi.org/10.4135/9781483391144.n166
17. Kolk, V. B. der, MD. (2015). *The body keeps the score: Brain, mind, and body in the healing of trauma* (Reprint). Penguin Publishing Group.
18. Smith, A. (2017). Introduction: The revolution will not be funded. In INCITE! (Ed.), *The revolution will not be funded: Beyond the non-profit industrial complex*. Duke University. (Original work published 2006)
19. Williams, A. K., Owens, R., & Syedullah, J., PhD. (2016). *Radical dharma: Talking race, love, and liberation* (Illustrated). North Atlantic Books.
20. Belkin Martinez, D. (2014). The liberation health model: Theory and practice. In D. Belkin Martinez & A. Fleck-Henderson (Eds.), *Social justice in clinical practice: A liberation health framework for social work*. Routledge.
21. Lorde, A. (2004). An Interview: Audre Lorde and Adrienne Rich. In *Sister outsider*. The Crossing Press. (Original work published 1984)
22. Leiner, R., & Syedullah, J. (2023). The manual for liberating survival: Lesson I, how self-care matters as an embodied practice of abolition. In A. Crawley & R. Sirvent (Eds.), *Spirituality and abolition*. Common Notions.
23. Brown, S. (2022). *Refusing compulsory sexuality: A Black asexual lens on our sex-obsessed culture*. North Atlantic Books.
24. Harrison, D. L., & Laymon, K. (2021). *Belly of the beast: The politics of anti-fatness as anti-blackness*. North Atlantic Books.
25. Woodland, E., & Page, C. (2023). *Healing justice lineages: Dreaming at the cross-roads of liberation, collective care, and safety*. North Atlantic Books.
26. Belser, A., & Keating, A. (2022). A queer vision for psychedelic research: Past reck-onings, current reforms, and future transformations. In A. Belser, C. Cavnar, & B. Labate (Eds.), *Queering psychedelics: From oppression to liberation in psychedelic medicine*. Synergetic Press.
27. Ransby, B. (1995). *Black popular culture and the transcendence of patriarchal illu-sions* (B. Guy-Sheftall & T. Matthews, Eds.). The New Press.
28. Hassan, S. (2022). *Saving our own lives: A liberatory practice of harm reduction* (D. G. Lewis, Ed.). Haymarket Books.
29. Lorde, A. (2019). Uses of the erotic: The erotic as power. In A. M. Brown (Ed.), *Pleasure activism: The politics of feeling good*. AK Press. (Original work published 1984)
30. Williams, A. K., Owens, R., & Syedullah, J., PhD. (2016). *Radical dharma: Talking race, love, and liberation* (Illustrated). North Atlantic Books.

Chapter 6

Cultural Evolution

Seeing Clearly

You can breathe. Memorizing historical context or understanding every societal expectation is not the aim of this offering. It is actually to destabilize your neo-cortex and make space for some emotions and sensations to take center stage, and to feel into the impossible nature of being able to grasp this all. It is actually to be with the is-ness of how little power, control, understanding we have. At any given single moment, there are multiple lenses we can regard that moment through or elements that are contributing to that moment. And even if we are well versed in a lens or an element, our understanding is not universal. It is not for everyone; it's not even true. It's what we have in that moment, and it is what we will use. Holding that tension is occupying an anti-oppressive seat.

To have an anti-oppressive therapeutic practice and seat, you need the capacity to look at what is not possible for the person in front of you, and you can do this by studying what is readily available and how it obstructs the capacity to see what else is possible. These obstructions can come from deep-held beliefs generated from their family of origin or from the social norms that they are being compared to, but also what is not possible because you, the therapist, do not possess the spaciousness for endless possibility. Our narrow view itself can be an obstruction to the possibilities available to a client working with us. These norms that are upheld by institutions, systems and families reside in us, too, the clinician. These norms that serve to benefit the wealth of the elites and who have little to no intention of bettering our lives, only that of their legacy, dictate our work. And to do something different, to offer a different experience, we have to look really widely; we must painfully acknowledge the contradictions within ourselves and how hiding them keeps us narrowly focused.

Contradictions in this culture are seen as a momentary state, we believe. That with time and effort, one side of the contradiction will be proven true. But actually, the world is made up of contradictions, and so are we. Contradictions are misaligned with the analytical framework that says everything should have a place and make sense. So it is deeply disruptive to neocortical supremacy to

DOI: 10.4324/9781003207054-8

allow and seek contradictions. Contradictions do not mean one of them is wrong; it actually is an invitation to explore how both can be true.

We will be unable to begin the process of truly imagining liberation for ourselves and our clients until we face all we dare not engage with in fear it contradicts something we know. When we go towards the contradictions, it leads us to seek clarity and, in there, opens up an opportunity to surrender to the truth that we may never fully understand. Through that surrendering we are able to make space for the unimaginable. So, this is an invitation to begin a lifelong practice of utilizing the expanded consciousness and access to knowledge of these times and widen our lens to include all the unknowns, all the invisible, all the mystery and surrender to awe.

So we have traveled through all of these realms which make up the elements that inform the anti-oppressive practice I am offering. When receiving a client who comes in with an issue they want resolved or a way of being that they are ready to retire or a desire they cannot meet, we want to honor their reasons for coming in while keeping in mind the broader context in which these reasons exist. Having this lens means we can see the importance of the issue they bring as it relates to the client, but also that this client is part of a bigger story and their issue tells us something about the collective and informs the collective. This additional frame I am promoting towards the client issue is how we embody the quote popularized and credited to Lilla Watson, who has said it is a product of indigenous wisdom and not her own: "If you have come here to help me, you are wasting your time. If you have come because your liberation is bound up with mine, then let us work together."[1]

The Anti-Oppressive Lens

That quote, although often used in a human-centered manner, is an entryway to an understanding of the biological term sympoietic. Sympoiesis is invoked when discussing organisms of differing species or types "becoming with" each other.[2] Becoming with simply means they cannot become themselves without each other. Or, they are themselves because of the other. I think we can borrow that sense to understand the anti-oppressive lens and its elements. It is the lens that looks to hold all of these elements when approaching another being, a situation, a moment. The elements are sympoietic. A non-human-centered example of attention to sympoiesis includes the plant life that is around your home. I sometimes find myself walking on the boardwalk near my home and I notice the plants growing. I often use an app on my phone to help me identify the plant. Immediately, my mind goes to wonder if this plant is native or was it imported and forcefully grown here. I wonder if the Canarsee people of Lenapehoking used this plant for medicine. I wonder if it has spiritual meaning. I usually go down a Google wormhole to learn if the plant would be medicine for any ailments of mine (real or perceived). When I see on my app a plant is considered a weed, I enjoy the plant more because it is deemed useless by capitalism. I wonder what kind of offering I would need to leave to take it home. And then, oftentimes, I just leave it as I found it so that it will be available for another traveler in the future. I wonder how it is shifting the air right now. I try to notice if my breathing changes in proximity to the plant. I consider if my closeness is giving it life, giving carbon dioxide. I wonder if it attracts or repels bugs, I fear. So on and so forth . . .

This seemingly unimportant exploration of my long-winded musings is why, as a young person, I was called a party pooper, or Debbie downer or one of my favorite people on social media, Ericka Hart's, Twitter handle: "Your fave killjoy."[3] I could not just let a thing be. I wanted to understand how I should interact with things, what was needed, and I could not know without a series of questions and evidence. I realize now I was trying to understand relatedness. I had an inclination that in all relationships, expectations should change, and so I needed to thoroughly understand the relationship to understand how I am to relate in it and how things are related to each other. And, in a culture that wants non-stop fun, excitement and good moods, my questions often do the opposite and ruin the mood (because good times in this culture rely on cognitive dissonance). Relatedness and sympoiesis are kind of my chicken and egg debate. Is something happening because it is responding to something else, or is it how it is with this other thing?

That is this lens. Having attention on the relatedness. Being with relatedness is a limbic exercise. This is not our culture. We are in a culture that reinforces dispositionalism. That there should be a systemized and generalized way of understanding and responding. Practicing attention to relatedness and increasing a sense of sympoiesis means looking and noticing, especially in places where it seems already buttoned up. It means to look for how what I experience is related to what has been hidden and what was made available to be seen. Practice includes a commitment to making the invisible, the unsaid, the assumed visible. I especially want us in this field to embrace this lens when we are serving other humans. If I can spend five minutes in front of the seaside goldenrod trying to understand how I should relate to it, I hope we are fully enthralled in this process with the people we serve.

When looking at the graph below, think of your lens right now as the anti-oppressive lens that can take in and consider all of these elements and their relationships to each other. Although they seem to include each other, they do not have to. Remember, as a culture steeped in and sustained by neocortical supremacy, we are oriented towards a narrow focus rather than a holistic view. So, although they all stand alone, they are actually all impacted by the others. An anti-oppressive lens does not mean mastering all of these elements; it is impossible. The lens *does* mean having a curiosity about the others no matter where you find your initial focus.

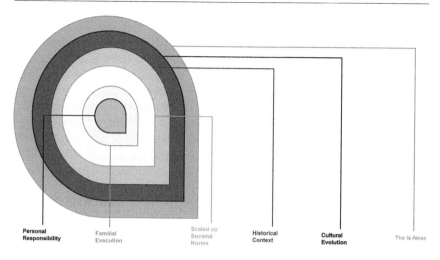

Personal Responsibility   Familial Execution   Scaled up Societal Norms   Historical Context   Cultural Evolution   The Is-Ness

Figure 6.1 An attempt to illustrate the anti-oppressive lens.

Feel Into It

I am going to make some generalizations in the next few pages that are mostly done in humor but I have had enough interactions with them to see how prevalent they are. You may have strong responses; again, that is a good noticing and probably where some unraveling can happen! Remember that from where I sit, in my identities, experiences and lens, this is how they appear to me. That is information for you.

What feels familiar here? How does it feel where you are seated? What does it feel like when you meet an edge/discomfort/upset? Where is there heartbreak and hopelessness? How does your body experience those emotions?

The point is to let yourself relate to these elements. Notice where they exist in you. Maybe your stomach lurches at some point; your legs shake at another. Maybe you notice your breath changes depth at a word or feel sudden exhaustion at another word. Track that.

All of the elements we will move through are present in all matters and moments. The tone with which I describe them is to highlight the narrow focus each element can have when exclusively utilized to understand a moment or material.

Personal Responsibility

This element is easily encountered and readily available in our society and our industry/field. Practitioners looking at the people they serve exclusively through this lens have fully embraced that individuation is a natural progression of life. In this realm, individual choice is the focus, the cause of suffering, and has the power to make a better life. In this element, the norms are not in question; the ability to adhere to them is. Here, they will interpret the client as the main factor in addressing their issue, becoming who they want to be or getting what they want. When using this element exclusively to understand the world, everyone is responsible for their own plight and our job is to redirect them. Although practitioners here may understand that everything is not fair, or we have been impacted by other elements, ultimately, it returns to the individual to override these setbacks, it is about willingness to put in the work. Whether it is cognitive or behavioral it is about putting in the work of changing your thoughts or feelings. This also applies to our new-age spiritualism, which is about attracting what you want hard enough for its manifestation. Toxic positivity and its practitioners definitely live in this domain. The idea that thinking good things determines what happens to them. It also uplifts the belief that if you are willing to work hard enough, you deserve what you get.

Here, emotions are fully inside a person and, therefore, able to be controlled by a person. Although there might be embodiment utilized, it is often in the service of gaining control over oneself. Someone working exclusively with this element agrees that there is normal human development; its goal is to be happy and healthy.

This lens is necessary in the anti-oppressive toolbox because, for the most part, that is what people expect from us. They expect insight and tools. They expect that we, too, want them to be happy.[4] Without it, we are bypassing how and why many clients enter therapy. Looking for relief from some suffering. It is also the element we are most familiar with ourselves if we were born and raised in the West, but also if we were educated in Western ideals. I am clear with my clients that I am not interested much in this element, and, for some people, they choose to find someone who is. This element has colluded with the idea that bodies are machines. That everything can be calculated. They may rely on chrononormativity, healthism and epistemic justice as guides in how to approach their work. A simple "if something is wrong, fix it" attitude can be taken. With enough experience "fixing" people, places and things, the clinician can rely on their competence and formulas and less on the client they are currently sitting across.

Staying here can seem very safe because it does rely on the clinician's sense of competence. It does not ask our limbic system to join; we stay neocortex-heavy and cognitively laborious. It is culture-aligned – that hard work is how we purify ourselves. It aligns with how we have been conditioned to understand ourselves and the world around us. It requires the least amount of disruption of our performance. Think about how quickly if you tell a friend you have an issue and they reply with, "Have you tried . . .?" That is how common this element is in our way of understanding how to support others.

In this realm, the client and practitioner will create a goal where they can measure their failure to meet it, or their success rate. This is the ideal lens for insurance-governed clinics, or venture-capitalist-backed psychedelic-assisted psychotherapy. It can be timed. It can be objectively evaluated and it protects systems. The practitioner also gets to protect themselves from being impacted by the client. This also ignores that humans are deeply inter-relational animals and that whether a client is choosing to please the therapist or their boss instead of their overbearing parent or problematic partner, they are still responding to a relationship. In this role, the therapist does not have to consider that they are in a relationship with the client where the client is looking to give the therapist what they want and vice versa. This is definitely where my pain came from when mourning RL. This lens is also a good way to get some easy wins because we live in a world where easy wins motivate us. I utilize this when I am seeing a client, and we have had a few difficult sessions or a few weeks of intensity. Or on days I cannot visit someone else's world because of the conditions of my own. I will offer a session where we get to stay neocortex to neocortex. I also will flow in and out of focusing on this element in a session. It is not shallow; it's simply not counter-cultural or limbically focused.

This lens does not pay attention to the backstage. It is more dealing with the performance. Remember that the performance is strategic; it is curated to meet societal expectations as executed by the family unit, medical system and all other managing institutions. This lens does not interrupt cognitive dissonance or Fundamental Attribution Error – it strengthens them. It is based on what performance the client wants to project that is in alignment with societal values and actually involves perfecting that performance. There is little room for conflictual information or opposing needs that may reside in the individual (client or practitioner). This leads to an increase to what belongs and is placed backstage. Although confession is used to seemingly address the backstage, we have seen how it actually strengthens the need for a backstage. It remains neocortically led, creating more strategy to respond to inconsistencies and uphold the idea of an individual autopoietic (self-generating) self. Because we are a culture run on neocortical performances that we cling to, as practitioners, we cannot dismiss this element; maintaining the skills to navigate this element is very important. Allowing people to have some of what they believe they need gives confidence, pride and actually may allow some detaching from the need to perform with a therapist, who is being watchful of the client's attachment to their performance and is offering limbic resonance opportunities and invitations to shift habitual performance. This element can be skillfully toggled and supportive when used in combination with the other elements.

Feel Into It

How does this section land in you?

Practice to Intervention

Read through this facetious case study. Then do your practice one below. Have fun with it. Compare with your reading group. Act some of it out, make sure to keep feeling yourself as you go along.

Problem: My stomach hurts. I have been overeating the last few weeks. It's because I am stressed.

Personal Responsibility: I should create a food journal that will remind me when to eat.

Personal Responsibility: I should keep only healthy foods in the house, so if I do overeat, I will eat good foods at least.

Personal Responsibility: I should go on the latest fad diet because it is different than the others and has worked wonders for some random person.

Personal Responsibility: I will do some other self-care activities to take care of my stress, and then I will naturally eat less.

Personal Responsibility: Go to the doctor and see if there is a hormonal issue happening causing this.

Your Turn:

Problem: Amare lives alone in a big city in the United States. They have been feeling very alone.

Personal Responsibility:

Familial Execution

Familial execution is the lens that looks to understand how the client, issue that needs solving, way of being that is not working, or elusive desire was influenced by personal history. Without actively thinking about it, we are often evaluating how the family executed their role as society recruiters. In this element, there is more acceptance that the individual is impacted by their environment and less desire to blame a client for their predicament, so there is some movement away from individual-centered autopoiesis. However, there is a belief in the autopoiesis of the family and genetics. Working exclusively with this element, the emphasis may be made on the brain, genetics, family of origin and their personal history.

Here, there is an attention to beliefs and looking for "root" causes. Practitioners may have a lot of interest in understanding the family of origin and maybe even with genealogy, bringing in some version of ancestral inheritance and intergenerational trauma. We might be very interested in supporting a client to understand their issues, behaviors and desires in response to the context they developed in. When used with somatics, it may be to support the client to return to the body. Here, the therapist may utilize their relationship with the client with the intention of being a presence that was missing in a client's childhood. A practitioner may look to engage and use their limbic system in their work, but without the wider lens, is unaware of how much more conditioning there is in their system that impacts the quality of their resonance. Although the practitioner may encourage limbic connection in the client, they can do this without tuning into their own systems if they understand their work neocortically only (which becomes another performance). This shows a misunderstanding of limbic resonance and its value.

Importantly, more acknowledgment is made that people are not only individuals – we are impacted, and continuously so, by our experiences. I appreciate this element because it was where I wanted to work. I wanted so badly to replicate a missing loving presence for my clients, but I continuously did not know what to do with the rage I had towards the society that made the conditions they (we) were trapped in or be with their rage when it came towards me.

I often think about how inaccessible this lens is when working with people who have been conditioned to be disembodied. There are scales of disembodiment. Being in memory or the body has been very dangerous for many of us. And I have found that many of the practitioners who operate in this zone seem to think that the scale of disembodiment doesn't matter too much. Or don't seem to believe that cultural origins vary and influence disembodiment. Instead of recognizing that the person is on a scale of disembodiment, the practitioner may make it about the client's readiness. There is a deep belief about human nature that tells them that these scales do not matter because "every person just wants the same things." And giving them those things will override the relentless memory of past devastating experiences and ongoing cultural onslaught. Folks in this element use "human nature" to support norms.

When I am in rooms with these clinicians, which is often, things are chucked up to human nature often. And when they say this, they mean ways of being they find desirable, which are dictated by social norms. They love "calm" and "happy." The thing is, I do not have to look far to find people who do not consider human nature calm and happy. These ideas of human nature are based on norms phrased as entitlements or rights and liberties. I suspect that these clinicians are only seeing clients who have had the same orientation as themselves in this culture. Because that human nature crap would shatter fast with some of the people I have worked with. I fear that when they are seeing other clients of differing backgrounds or orientations towards the world, they are using their power position to implicitly imply that their idea of human nature is correct; therefore, the clients perceived limitations are wrong. The practitioners stuck in this way of being have no desire to interrupt this delusion in themselves, so they definitely cannot interrupt it anywhere else. I think about how many student clinicians or new clinicians run away from the clients and communities they are trained in, for clients who are "ready" for their skillset. In other words, clients who are "calmer" and do not have any external needs that require their attention, clients who "can turn inward." Those clients they prefer are often those who have benefited from societal values and have been rewarded with financial compensation that allows them to afford a therapist who "gets it." I've also seen how this approach has been used to dismiss, gaslight and infantilize people's experiences.

I have found the people here are fine to witness anger when it is towards your mother, who is not in the room, than to have it come towards them. The preference for calm and orderly also protects the fragility and worldview of the therapist. That there are certain ways your body should feel, there are certain feelings that are good and if it hadn't been for your absent mom, or your family being poor or your sexual assault, you would have been normal. Here, in many ways, we are saying, "I believe you, that event did make you abnormal, but I think with enough care, attention and support we can get you closer to normal again." This is the opposite of sympoiesis.

In this element, there is an idea that we will return to the original you that was unscathed by trauma. That even under all the parts that are looking to protect you, there is a pure part.[5] First, I argue that our culture is traumatic. Ignoring our culture allows us to focus on individual incidents rather than the consistent and ongoing threat to life that begins before birth in the West. Secondly, I do not hear seriously enough that there is no pureness. The essential self has been responding to their environment since in utero. This belief does not allow acceptance for who and what you are now; it is driven by "There is a better you somewhere, and our goal should be heading towards it."

Therapy done exclusively in this section can lean towards a goal of feeling good/better. These emotions are valued in our society, which can make our work towards them a performance-strengthening task. This task will explicitly engage cognitive dissonance to ignore conflicting information that threatens the fragility of "feeling good" (also see worthy, entitled, happy, proud, powerful and important). It can create another performance that protects backstage material, strengthening Fundamental Attribution Error, even if some backstage material surfaces through confession. A clinician who has not done their own limbic remembering and grieving will use neocortical strategies and miss the conflictual and non-easily categorized experiences present to attend to. They will aim to clean things up, not swim in the mess of things.

Feel Into It

How does this section land in you?

Practice to Intervention

Read through this facetious case study. Then do your practice one below. Have fun with it. Compare with your reading group. Act some of it out, make sure to keep feeling yourself as you go along.

Problem: My stomach hurts. I have been overeating the last few weeks. It's because I am stressed.

Familial Execution: Growing up, food was such a reliable comfort for me, and it's ok to use it for comfort in times of stress. We all deserve comfort; it's our right.

Familial Execution: When I am stressed, I go to my happy place. My happy place is an imaginary/visualization of a beach.

Familial Execution: Food is such an important part of Haitian culture, and I should respect that.

Familial Execution: I work with my therapist to notice the sensations of wanting to eat in my body and learn that it is really my anxiety that is causing me to feel pain.

Your Turn:

Problem: Amare lives alone in a big city in the United States. They have been feeling very alone.

Familial Execution:

Scaled-Up Societal Norms

Here is where I think most people who call themselves anti-oppressive work from. This element is filled with the unavoidable injustice that makes life so damn difficult! The injustices are results of the conditions that have been created out of scaling up societies with a focus on increasing power through wealth. These are folks who hold a social analysis very valuable to their practice. They are taking into account institutional and systemic influences on the lives of individuals. They are often addressing individual suffering by challenging the systems that benefit from that suffering. They often support clients to see themselves as more normal in that there are more people who are in their situation than those who have achieved "societal norms."

Clinicians who operate exclusively from here might have a goal of supporting the client to remember themselves as a powerful member "of the people." This is where social justice as healing work would come into play. Looking to regain power for the individual by connecting them to the "powerful" mass. The goals in this element may be about connecting to righteous anger. Anger in our culture is a better feeling than sad because anger means there is still "a claim for dominance,"[4] and dominance is good. See, although we use the language "freedom," progressive movements since the creation of world-economy systems and the concept of citizens, most movements were about being accepted as a citizen, about inclusion within oppressive systems.[6] These movements for inclusion mean there is alignment with the illusion of superiority the perceived oppressors have. Working from this place exclusively may dismiss the individual hurt and pain by these structures that impact families and harm individuals. Having these feelings may be seen as resignation or unuseful in getting what is "owed." Somehow, although this realm is all about pushing back against powers of oppression, it often uses similar tactics, such as seeing individuals as collectibles for their scaling-up agenda, that individuals can be data points that predict the future, that bodies are machines that can be worked to purity. I have been a client and have worked with clients who reside here who felt if we allowed ourselves to be heartbroken, we would stop being useful to the movement, and usefulness is where our sense of belonging is coming from.

What also happens here is we externalize our anger and hide that being raised or educated in these ideals comes with the same indoctrination we are fighting against. Here, it seems easier to focus on external harms rather than recognize how we have internalized them.[7] Practitioners here may not take into account how these theories are intellectual, and they lack embodiment or practice. I have been in psychedelic-assisted guided sessions and fought rest. Seeing my body's need for rest as a betrayal, afraid of some deep, dark part of myself that would stop me from being a "soldier for the good side." This keeps our attention, energy and life force focused on a conceptual belonging as opposed to actual belonging. All of this is directly linked to the false idea of there being a powerful yet dormant mass. It also utilizes that my life needs purpose or meaning to the collective to be worth living. This is not very different from the elites' beliefs of the masses. Many of the strategies and tactics utilized replicate the strategies used for oppression. Here, we think we are making space but end up policing each other with political correctness and virtue signaling, encouraging more performance.[8]

I used to happily stay focused on the scaled-up society expectation element. And because I could blame others outside of myself, I did not see how I utilized personal responsibility as a motivator. It also meant it was years before I was able to really see how my familial relationships have impacted me. Remember from my introduction that I was consumed with an anger and rage that kept me up at night and pushed away the hopelessness I felt. I would say this narrow lens is how organizers can perpetuate abusive behaviors while working to "free us all." That oppression is not simply an intellectual matter; it has been reinforced generationally and personally more than our desire to not be oppressed.

Sadly, success in these worlds mirror capitalism; they still value scaling up, increasing reach, breaking up kinship bonds for voluntary organizations, creating norms around behavior, thoughts, language and health that must be adhered to for the members to remain in connection. Success still looks like being able to be the one who dictates what is normal, substituting surveilling inner thoughts for surveilling language. I used to organize Clinicians in NYC through Radical Social Worker Group[9] and within that Clinical Workgroup, and there were, and still are, many Social Workers (including myself) who burned out regularly who work primarily with this element. They were working to support clients, pushing against the policy of their institutions and work culture, organizing and marching on the weekends and evenings. Consumed with reading and learning and very often internalized the "never good" enough drive. These folks are also working an impossible task that will never be satiated and allow rest and presence. This keeps a future-focused perpetual motion, which is very neocortical. Here, "we dehumanize ourselves in our practice of becoming workaholics for the movement. We are competitive about how busy we are in advancing it."[10]

This is not a blanket statement because I have also heard in the Healing Justice world, people who are spiriting that embodiment must come along with analysis, so must spirit, so must connection. I got to witness this in the Healing Justice Learning and Strategy Lab curated and facilitated by the National Queer And Trans Therapists Of Color Network[11]. Also, reading *Radical Dharma: Talking Race, Love and Liberation* (mentioned in Chapter 1) and *Healing Justice Lineages: Dreaming at the Crossroads of Liberation, Collective Care, and Safety*[12] by Cara Page and Erica Woodland has shown me the other possibilities for holding the analysis of our position and accepting and caring for others as they are. They collude with possibility. "Our work is to invent and imagine healing that increases both individual options and interrupts systemic harms."[13] These folks are not exclusively using this element, though; there is a combination happening that allows for this type of spaciousness and wide view.

Working from this lens exclusively is all neocortex all the time. Without explicit attention to bring in limbic, backstage, complicated, contradictory material, therapists here may strengthen cognitive dissonance. Which is ironic because so many of these therapists are committed to shattering social cognitive dissonance. Without attention on what moral values they are "replacing" social ones with, they may swap one dissonance for another, giving a new set of ways of being that must be stored in an expanded backstage. Fundamental Attribution Error is also maintained, sometimes swapping out one consistent performance for another. Often creating our own new set of social rules. These rules may actually continue to isolate and disembody us. The therapist here would need to have those shattered as well and grieved the cultural value of disconnection limbically to feel the difference in values. From this felt understanding, they may create the small-scale change that can satisfy themselves and the place, land, people and non-human beings they belong to. The idea that sticking to new values over relationships is a recreation of disconnection.

This element can also be quite mechanistic and autopoietic. The attention may move away from being with our limbic need for each other, sometimes even exploiting that need. From this approach, we end up using each other rather than sharing with and in each other, which Audre Lorde warns against in *Uses of the Erotic*. We may think our mission is more important than relationships and encourage that in clients.

Feel Into It

How does this section land in you?

Practice to Intervention

Read through this facetious case study. Then do your practice one below. Have fun with it. Compare with your reading group. Act some of it out, make sure to keep feeling yourself as you go along.

Problem: My stomach hurts. I have been overeating the last few weeks. It's because I am stressed.

Scaled-Up Societal Norms: This anti-fat culture is the reason I am judging my eating. I need to know that the average American is closer to my size than the average supermodel.

Scaled-Up Societal Norms: It's the goal of the oppressor I die early, so I should get a handle on this to be useful to the mission.

Scaled-Up Societal Norms: The ingredients in overly processed foods are meant to make us addicted and return for more. We need to look at the food industry.

Scaled-Up Societal Norms: There is a community farm that delivers healthy foods to people in need; maybe volunteer there and start mending my relationship to food.

Scaled-Up Societal Norms: I should go to the next rally; nothing relieves stress like screaming in the streets.

Your Turn:

Problem: Amare lives alone in a big city in the United States. They have been feeling very alone.

Scaled-Up Societal Norms:

Historical Context

This element looks towards the practitioners that look to history to inform the present. Here, we may glorify the rituals, rites and traditions of a historic society. I use the word glorify because there is a feeling that how it was done before was correct and that there is no access to that now. These are people who are looking to history for insight into how to navigate our current times. The goal may be to have a "simpler life" that takes away all the pain of the times. I would place my spiritual bypassers here. This focus on historical events might increase the dissociation that helps shield from the pain of the times.[14]

I find that people exclusively working with this element idolize the past and whitewash it. They decontextualize history, making it spontaneous and stuck in time. It does not take into account that the conditions of the current time differ greatly and that rituals, rites and traditions have always and must always respond to and meet the challenges and needs of the times. Taking practices from other cultures, also known as appropriation, is not a form of flattery; it is a form of erasure.[15] Again, here I pull up Western psychedelic practitioners who enjoy the title of shaman or another such title, completely taking and using other cultural practices, ignoring the power differential that was present when they got "initiated" in another practice or they took what was not meant for them. Here, they still see other cultures as primitive and less human, even if it is placing them on a pedestal of divine or closer to natural. They often are inadvertently implying "the role of indigenous people is reduced to their historical function as preservers of these practices until they can be 'discovered' by more sophisticated people better able to understand and explain them."[16]

There is often a desire for a simpler time when, in fact, no time recorded in history seems simple. They may want to encourage their clients to pull away from the current world for one constructed out of cognitive dissonance and disassociation. "There is in this hatred of the present or the immediate past a dangerous tendency to invoke a completely mythical past."[17] It does not address the pain and grief of not having the kinship or relationship to land or other beings that made the rituals so powerful and supportive. Without incorporating that history, you decontextualize whole cultures, making them spontaneous rather than the ongoing experience they are. Without the context, we cannot be aware of how we are continuing the separation from ourselves by ignoring the current context we are in. We need the lived experience of this moment to know the rituals and rites necessary to traverse this time.

Understanding how the ancient Greeks interpreted the moon does not inform us on how we have been conditioned to understand the moon. Those beliefs were informed by the times and evolved from other traditions because they were sympoietic – "becoming with" with non-human, the elements, nature and humans. We also must be able to see how our lenses are doomed to misinterpret and make things make sense to us. I highly recommend reading *Post Colonial Astrology: Reading the Planets through Capital, Power and Labor*[18] by Alice Sparkly Kat to get a fantastic view into how easily we convert history to match our lens and misuse tradition. That how we see the moon is literally different than how it was seen then and there. Foucault warns, "[Y]ou can't find the solution of a problem in the solution of another problem raised at another moment by other people."[19] You can be inspired, yes, you can envy, sure, but you cannot swap it in. So much of historical interpretation is inaccessible to us because of the very different psychologies of the people, place and times we are looking for. It is like we are plucking out a favorable part of history and completely erasing the realities of that time and its incongruency with this time. This element viewed exclusively usually returns to personal responsibility, ignoring the real barriers to the well-being of people in the West.

Listen, I also live here. I have so many herbs at any given moment to make a variety of teas to support me with a variety of maladies that are totally foreign to the land I inhabit. I have adopted a devotional practice to Kuan Yin Bodhisattva that is not from my culture. I love a ritual! I use them to regularly connect with spirit along with many divination tools. I have a daily yoga and chanting practice, get acupuncture, frequent deprivation tanks, and have psychedelic medicine journeys. Utilizing all these borrowed technologies and traditions to make me feel better has been beautiful, and still, I know the privilege I had to quit my job helped me with stress more than any of those put together. I know the privilege I had to move to the beach away from the middle of Brooklyn calmed my nervous system more than any of those practices. I know the space and time I have to practice my rituals support their potency. So, simply taking them out of context is not the medicine alone. They are helpful, they are my lifeline and they cannot override the oppression that is on attack every day. We have to be with the contradictions within ourselves in our practices.

Practitioners exclusively focused in this element increase cognitive dissonance. History and what we steal from history, like spiritual practices, can be used to escape current conditions. They may swap out which "truths" they want to see, but there will be a lot of the present conditions that conflict with their truths and must be ignored and denied. Practitioners may use their neocortex to understand limbic needs, but without their own shattering and grieving of reality, they will encourage Fundamental Attribution Error because they have strong beliefs in what is right and wrong ways to be which individuals are asked to adhere to. There may be more of a desire to live sympoietically, but without looking at Western human supremacy and neocortical supremacy, they will ultimately continue to assist the Anthropocene. There often is a nostalgia for a community of a mythical past that appears sympoietic (think commune) but must be extracted from the complex, real society in which we exist.

Our cultural evolution has overcomplicated survival and our psychology. Anti-oppressive is not making believe that there is some better place out there; it is more about being willing to look at why this place cannot be that place. Not in an effort to make it that place but to be with the clarity of the place, time, space we exist in. "Anything aboriginal that enters the artificial space of Western culture is diminished, changed to fit into it," warns Somé.[17]

I am often disturbed by the amount of gaslighting that happens here, making it about individual faith or belief rather than literal barriers created by society. This is a major concern I have about the psychedelic industry in its new iteration. We ignore its lineage is not traditional Indigenous use. The history of psychedelics in the colonized West is based on the values of Western psychology and the field of psychiatric medicine.[20] We are selling people the idea of magic, and for many of us, magical experiences happen, but our lives outside the magic are often what we are "becoming with." We need to hold both in equanimity. Not place one as a more superior or right experience.

The issue with exclusively residing in the element of historical context is that it is resigned; it is like throwing the baby out with the bath water. It does not believe that this time we are in can offer anything to alleviate suffering. It does not believe in the power of ending the Anthropocene and becomes consumed with an individual living a peaceful life, despite it all.

Feel Into It

How does this section land in you?

Practice to Intervention

Read through this facetious case study. Then do your practice one below. Have fun with it. Compare with your reading group. Act some of it out, make sure to keep feeling yourself as you go along.

Problem: My stomach hurts. I have been overeating the last few weeks. It's because I am stressed.

Historical Context: These are herbs the Canarsee people used to help calm them when they were activated. I can drink this tea to help me lessen my body's stress.

Historical Context: I can join a women's circle that meets regularly to help the body find its "natural" rhythm; in matrilineal societies, this was how the culture survived.

Historical Context: In Chinese medicine, they use acupuncture to regulate stress and curb hunger; I should try that.

Historical Context: In many cultures before anti-blackness, having weight was seen as a sign of wealth. I should move proudly.

Your Turn:

Problem: Amare lives alone in a big city in the United States. They have been feeling very alone.

Historical Context:

Cultural Evolution

It bears a constant reminder that cultural evolution is not innovation. It is the ongoing cultural shifts in response to a society's history, location and norms through subtle competition. Not active competition as in "ready, set, go," competition as in these norms are more likely to generate and sustain what a society values. Cultural evolution is where I do not counter enough in this field. It is the understanding that there is such a thing as a collective consciousness that breeds new cultural norms while diminishing old ones. It is an unintentional movement. For some cultures and societies, cultural evolution is slow and the needs of the society are continually met by their practices. In the West, cultural evolution is faster, since a value of this society is innovation.

In the West, cultural evolution must take into account the historical underpinnings of norms and values of the time to understand the emergence of an omnipresent and punishing god. It needs to feel the separation from kinship-based networks as a strategy to please this god. It needs to understand how the values of growth and scaling up that came from centuries of shifts in collective consciousness created these huge societies and made individualization a norm. These huge societies prioritized order and control to maintain power over other societies, which created governments. These governments outsourced their value of order, control and discipline to hospitals, doctors, prisons and police. These professionals created norms through "science" that were used to evaluate families. These families attempted to adhere to these norms and raise children according to them on their own. Everyone in a family had to be personally responsible for themselves to make it work. Cultural value cannot be seen exclusive of the preceding elements. It is taking into account the historical context that made our societal expectations necessary that were executed by the families and the personal responsibilities dictated to each individual in this culture.

Cultural evolution is not about placing blame or avoiding responsibility; it is about seeing change as being the only constant. It is about recognizing change will happen and how change happens is based on all of the other elements. Cultural evolution in another culture looks very different. Cultural evolution of an immigrant in the West looks different. Cultural evolution of devalued identities such as Black people, Indigenous people or Trans people in the West looks different. However, cultural evolution can hold the conflicting truth that at this point in time, white Westerners' cultural evolution has impacted all of those because their evolution idealizes dominance through the erasure of others.

Cultural evolution is where the collective is not something to blame, nor is it something to fix; it is something to regard as a living organism. This extends to the individual. Seeing it as a living organism means every interaction we have, every story we hear, every beautiful thing we witness and every heartbreaking news we are told is part of the organism and is informing us of where we are. Cultural evolution is echolocating. It is using what is around us to locate ourselves. Seeing ourselves as a product of many relationships. It shifts hearing clients from telling separate stories of personal incidents, but an offering of valuable puzzle pieces. And if we investigate ourselves, we'll find those pieces in us, too. It is all information. Cultural evolution requires that practitioners can tolerate contradiction. More than tolerate, they must seek it, including contradiction of feelings, of nature, of morality. Because it is all totally made up, so it can be demolished, we can destroy it, we can even leave it, but wherever we go, it'll still be in us. Whatever practices we try to appropriate to make us feel we are not of this culture are taken in the form of this culture. An anti-oppressive seat lives here, right in this tension. Knowing there is an is-ness that we may never encounter. We see the collective, want freedom for the collective, know the truth that our shackles are made up and yet, it lives in us.

Be wary, this is also where resignation occurs. The feeling of "What's the point?" The difference between resignation and acceptance must be clear. Acceptance does not stop us from looking. Resignation may turn us away from taking in new experiences. These fine lines need much attention. Cultural evolution is not taking the easy way out. It is about letting things be complicated, nuanced and confusing. Having conflicting ideas reside in the same statement. Cultural evolution can look like a long back-and-forth where nothing cancels another out, only widens the view and clarifies the scene.

Practitioners here are actively using the neocortex to give up its control and allow the limbic system to teach about sympoiesis. Cultural evolution is a human-centered yet wide-view sympoiesis. This lens helps break up our reliance on analysis and logic so that we can surrender to the realness of being bodies, animals, beings dependent on a variety of other bodies, animals and beings. Practitioners, anti-oppressive ones, can hold conflict and tension of truths, so are often looking to disillude themselves of cognitive dissonance. They are very aware that change is the constant and strive to disentangle themselves from Fundamental Attribution Error. This makes the backstage and performance sympoietic, that they become with each other. This adjustment allows the practitioner working here to invite them to integrate. Culturally, when we say integrate, we are often actually thinking of domination. Domination such as merge, when one entity actually outcompetes and overpowers the other and forces themselves into oneness. Here, I mean integrate as in both exist together because they are because the other one is.

Feel Into It

How does this section land in you?

Practice to Intervention

Read through this facetious case study. Then do your practice one below. Have fun with it. Compare with your reading group. Act some of it out, make sure to keep feeling yourself as you go along.

Problem: My stomach hurts. I have been overeating the last few weeks. It's because I am stressed.

Cultural Evolution: I am stressed because I need to complete this book. I have to finish this book because I made a time-bound commitment. I made a time-bound commitment because that is how contracts work in the West; fake rules to maintain forward movement. Food has always been a comfort for me and I have felt much shame about that. Being healthy is a made-up concept created so that I can be productive. This is not even my lineage as my family is not from this culture, yet I learned and internalized this historical background through my schooling, upbringing as Catholic and media. And due to the colonization and destabilization done by the United States of my parents' homeland, they have taken on these norms as superior. So, this judgment I am feeling towards myself is from a made-up standard, but I still believe in it. I am angry that I have internalized these views; I feel I should be better than this; here comes shame again. Although being healthy is made up, there are social consequences I will suffer for being overweight and not finishing the book. This is a frustrating bind I keep finding myself in. And my stomach is always hurting. I know I shouldn't, but I want to just ignore this and move on and get done what I need to do. I am going to drink that tea, though, and see if it will quiet my stomach until I have the space to figure out what is going on. All of this is true, and my stomach is still in pain. I will choose to just be with the sensation.

Your Turn:

Problem: Amare lives alone in a big city in the United States. They have been feeling very alone.

Cultural Evolution:

The Is-Ness

The is-ness is just what is.

I often see practitioners of different spiritual faiths believe they are here, but often after some conversation, I learn this is more aspirational and part of their performance, but their shadow run by backstage material shows what is not invited to exist and is far from being integrated. Since this culture strives for happiness, success and pride and avoids feelings of grief, shame and anger, it makes sense that bypassing happens so often here. Someone who attempts to exist exclusively in the is-ness is engaged in an addiction like any other; it eases the pain of reality with an escape route.

There is too much happening at any given moment to reside here. I'm sure some practitioner somewhere believes they do. But even our most enlightened ones fall out of this element and lens. It's filled with mystery and simplicity.

Feel Into It

How does this section land in you?

Practice to Intervention

Read through this facetious case study. Then do your practice one below. Have fun with it. Compare with your reading group. Act some of it out, make sure to keep feeling yourself as you go along.

Problem: My stomach hurts. I have been overeating the last few weeks. It's because I am stressed.

The Is-Ness: I am eating. The planet is turning. Things are dying. Things are being created. There is suffering. There is delight.

Your Turn:

Problem: Amare lives alone in a big city in the United States. They have been feeling very alone.

The Is-ness:

Final Note

None of the approaches to my issue were wrong or bad; they were simply incomplete without each other. An Anti-Oppressive Lens is taking all of this in. The overly complicated understanding that comes from cultural evolution and the simplicity of the is-ness. An anti-oppressive lens is sitting right between these conflicts and not needing either to go away. It is knowing much is out of our control, there is a lot that our good intentions and well wishes will not ease and all is as it should be.

I am not a "be the change you want to see in the world" person as we use it, which often means do something. I am a "feel the place you are in" person. The place you are in is in between seeing the change you want to see and it not being so. Bayo Akomolafe calls this "being in the cracks," and in this crack is grief.[21] What we continually fail to believe in this culture is that grief is generative; it carries with it its own medicine – possibility. Shame is medicine that brings with it longing for connection. Rage is a medicine that brings with it clarity. Sadly, we are not in a culture that teaches how to be in the crack. It is a foreign place for many of us. And worse than foreign, because we love foreign here in the West, we've been taught to believe that it is dangerous. But for many moments, it's actually unpleasant, not dangerous. Our connections between unpleasant and dangerous are interwoven here. And unpleasant we cannot do. Our entire worlds are built around making life comfortable, so we rarely seek the unpleasant, uncomfortable, the discordant, but we must because they lead to the crack where all that medicine is abundant and generous.

I love to run workshops where my goal is to make clinicians a bit uneasy, to feel doubt and less confident about what this work is we have chosen to do. One workshop I did earlier this year, a participant came up to me afterwards to share her experience of the meditation we did. In it, she described being in a mucky, gross, slimy and viscous swamp, and she saw herself swimming in it really feeling the disgust present, and then she realized she did not want to get out. She would rather be swimming in this mess than get out and do something else. I was moved to tears when I heard that; I felt like we found a crack to be in together. That is what is possible when we can be with. We can have these unpleasant and damn near disturbing experiences and not run or hide from them, but find a true unperformed space in ourselves that simply wants to still be on the journey.

There is something erotic about that choice, a different type of power. Something that belongs to just her, just us. It is sensual, this being with, it should be. It offers a different kind of agency which is not based on entitlements but based on personal power. We return to the uses of the erotic Audre Lorde left us.[15] The culture we are in, "the principal horror of such a system is that it robs our work of its erotic value, its erotic power and life appeal and fulfillment."[22] Anti-oppressive is grabbing that erotic power, that life appeal and fulfillment back from a sociopathic culture and embodying it, bathing ourselves in it, letting it drape all around us, swimming in it and allowing it to guide us.

Practice to Intervention

- Which lens do you rely on most?
- Which are you farthest from?

Share with your group. Create some intentions witnessed by each other. The intentions can include:

- What from my primary lens am I ready to retire?
- What in the aspirational lens am I looking to practice?
- What does practice look like?
- How can I be supported by the group in this pursuit?
- What do I have to offer someone in the group that struggles, where I find ease?

Citations

1. Original unknown.
2. Haraway, D. J. (2016). *Staying with the trouble: Making Kin in the Chthulucene (experimental futures)* (Illustrated). Duke University Press Books.

3. Your fave killjoy| Ericka Hart (she/they) (@iHartEricka)/. (2020, August 29). *Twitter*. https://twitter.com/ihartericka

4. Mesquita, B. (2022). *Between us: How cultures create emotions*. W. W. Norton & Company.

5. Kolk, V. B. der, MD. (2015). *The body keeps the score: Brain, mind, and body in the healing of trauma* (Reprint). Penguin Publishing Group.

6. Wallerstein, I. (2004). World-systems analysis. In *Duke University Press eBooks*. Duke University Press. https://doi.org/10.1215/9780822399018

7. Lorde, A. (2007). Eye to eye: Black women, hatred, and anger. In *Sister outsider*. The Crossing Press. (Original work published 1983)

8. Lorde, A. (2007). Learning from the 60s. In *Sister outsider*. The Crossing Press. (Original work published 1983)

9. Leiner, R., & Syedullah, J. (2023). The manual for liberating survival: Lesson I, how self-care matters as an embodied practice of abolition. In A. Crawley & R. Sirvent (Eds.), *Spirituality and abolition*. Common Notions.

10. Radical Social Work Group. (2019, December 27). *Closing a chapter*. Tumblr. https://radicalsocialworkgroup.tumblr.com/

11. Woodland, E. (2022). Home – national queer and trans therapists of color network. *National Queer & Trans Therapists of Color Network*. https://nqttcn.com/en/

12. Woodland, E., & Page, C. (2023). *Healing justice lineages: Dreaming at the crossroads of liberation, collective care, and safety*. North Atlantic Books.

13. Hassan, S. (2022). *Saving our own lives: A liberatory practice of harm reduction* (D. G. Lewis, Ed.). Haymarket Books.

14. Thanissara. (2015). *Time to stand up: An engaged Buddhist manifesto for our earth -- The Buddha's life and message through feminine eyes (sacred activism)* (1st ed.). North Atlantic Books.

15. Pagán, J. C. (n.d.). *Love and lightwashing: A guide to cultural appropriation, White privilege, and the shadow side of spirituality*. Spirit Guides Magazine.

16. Feinberg, B. (2018). Undiscovering the Pueblo Mágico: Lessons from Huautla for the psychedelic renaissance. *Plant Medicines, Healing and Psychedelic Science*, 37–54. https://doi.org/10.1007/978-3-319-76720-8_3

17. Somé, M. P. (1997). *Ritual: Power, healing and community (compass)* (1st ed.). Penguin Books.

18. Kat, S. A. (2021). *Postcolonial astrology: Reading the planets through capital, power, and labor*. North Atlantic Books.

19. Foucault, M., & Rabinow, P. (1984). *The Foucault reader*. Pantheon.

20. Brennan, B. P. (2020, August 11). *The revolution will not be psychologized: Psychedelics' potential for systemic change*. Chacruna. https://chacruna.net/the-revolution-will-not-be-psychologized-psychedelics-potential-for-systemic-change/

21. Akomolafe, B. (n.d.). We will dance with mountains: Into the cracks! In *https://course.bayoakomolafe.net/* [Course].

22. Lorde, A. (2019). Uses of the erotic: The erotic as power. In A. M. Brown (Ed.), *Pleasure activism: The politics of feeling good*. AK Press. (Original work published 1984)

Chapter 7

The Is-Ness Part II

Becoming Vulnerable

That erotic power described at the end of Chapter 6 is not easy to come into in this culture. It takes so much initial effort. What I hope is that I have made it alluring to try. That there is a spark of interest in this power and what it may offer rising in you. This power comes from what we've devalued and named feminine, the soft, the nurtured, the protected, the vulnerable. I want us to become vulnerable.

When I say vulnerable, I do not mean in the dismissive way we are towards non-power-grabbing feelings. Culturally, we are made to believe that if there is crying involved, it means someone is being vulnerable. That is a Fundamental Attribution Error; like everything else, crying is an expression that requires context to make sense of, it does not equal vulnerability. For example, in a group where there is often crying, it is actually the norm of that group. What might feel vulnerable in that group is someone saying, "I don't want to cry today. I feel like laughing." This person having to tolerate the unwanted desire in themselves and then taking the risk of sharing that with the group is vulnerable. This vulnerability is actually an invitation to the group to echolocate. For the group to accept that this person has something else in them that wants to be expressed, and the group gets to hold that, too. Let us work as therapists to separate tears and vulnerability, allowing one to be an emotional state and the other a bodily expression. Emotions and bodily expression such as crying are limbic experiences that we give meaning to with our neocortex that is created within this culture.

Vulnerability, being willing to share a need, want or experience and expecting it to be met, not fulfilled but met, is a courageous act in this culture. The capacity to meet someone's vulnerability is a huge task. Unfortunately, in the social service industry, we use "met" a lot but we do not mean it in the echolocating way I am hoping. We say things like "meet them where they're at," which has a seemingly good intention of beginning where the client is currently and not where you want them to be. I always felt torn about the phrase, and Shira Hassan clarified my discomfort perfectly; there is often an implication that we are meeting them

DOI: 10.4324/9781003207054-9

where they are at "so we can move them to where we think they should be."[1] This is not the type of "met" I mean. I mean met as in witnessed, held in regard, allowed to exist as is and embraced. When I say met, I mean as in "nothing is wrong with you." That experience of being met brings with it new possibilities. Those new possibilities occur in the body, the spirit, the limbic system, but the neocortical mind must come along to start.

The experience of meeting someone is also hard work. Because this is not an intellectual recognition; it is an embodied one that comes with sometimes "unpleasant" feelings. Often, these unpleasant feelings happen when something we are witnessing in another rubs against parts of us we have not sat with before. However, with personal practices of increasing our ability to be with our emotions and the sensations that express them, we can see our discomfort in right-proportion. It is not blown out to be a huge life-shattering experience that disconnects us from the moment. We can stay with our experience and still relate to that of another without having to diminish a part of them so we can stay with what is comfortable. Because "when we fail to relate to our own complexity, we fail to see the complexity of other people."[2] But when we are willing to be with complexity, it is a radical act. This is the work of collective shifting, cultural evolution contribution, because we are interrupting our training and tendency towards dissonance and instead choosing resonance.

So, to meet vulnerability, we must cultivate vulnerability. That is an anti-oppressive must.

Feel Into It

What happens in you when you hear a call to be vulnerable? Your gut, jaw, hands?

Practice to Intervention

What happens when you imagine it in relation to yourself? Your close relationships? Clients?

Right Proportion

Having an anti-oppressive seat means to place ourselves in the position to interrupt dispositionalism and the Anthropocene, to seek being in right-proportion as individuals and a species. Right-proportion means seeing things in their is-ness without bypassing reality. It is an ongoing quest to tear down the illusion of individuality by recognizing we are impacted and impacting at all times. To sense sympoiesis. To experience being a tiny part of a large organism called living. To feel de-centered and small. To disrupt neocortical supremacy so we can learn to trust our limbic system again. To be willing to be unimportant, unintelligent and confused. To put down our analysis and be holistic, see the full image, not just the target (especially when we are the target). To feel into the despair, grief and rage that is readily available in this place and look suspiciously at inclinations to jump over these for the sake of simplicity or politeness. To reach towards other humans and other non-human beings for their wisdom as a piece of the puzzle we need, to have a holistic view. To refuse to be veiled in what is easy but seek complicated. Right-proportion is knowing we cannot decontextualize a problem or a moment. In any moment, we can drop into the experience of the world, the experience in our bodies and the experience between beings. Right-proportion is knowing that there is more than we'll ever know. It is acceptance and even relief in the unknown and unknowable. We do this through unlearning and embodying ourselves. Occupying this seat is no easy task.

Quick detour. I find that people link right-proportion with this experience of oneness with the universe that people experience in orgiastic states like those in Psychedelic Assisted Psychotherapy in the West. Although there might be an is-ness truth to oneness with the universe, it is often not in right-proportion because "while substances may have common recognizable pharmacological effects on the human brain, these shared processes are interpreted in ways that are pro-foundly influenced and framed by culture, history and social relationships."[3] In other words our lens' interpret spirit. And often when I hear the oneness stories, I still hear an underpinning of "center of the universe" and/or "the chosen one." This grandiosity is still more likely to happen in this culture than in other cultural usage or in antiquity, where it would be more aligned with getting in right rela-tionships between warring clans, nature, ancestors and simply to build relation-ships with the plant.[4] For practitioners in this field, it is important we learn about historical and other cultural uses of these entheogens so we can detach them from the cultural expectations we place on them.

The grandiosity is demonstrated in the amount of people who have one experi-ence and realize they should be a facilitator too or open a clinic or save the world from itself. That is simply our culture. It doesn't mean that we don't do it, but we must take into account how culture plays a role in the entitlement that comes from these experiences. The visions may introduce the sense of sympoiesis, but the message is muddied because of our cultural lens that still looks to dominate, innovate and create individual identity and legacy. Right-proportion allows us to be with the experience without making it into validation of our entitlements.

What the Seat Is Not

An anti-oppressive seat is not about teaching clients about social inequities. Tell-ing clients, "Society is the problem, not you," is of very little use to them. It instead can dismiss their experience. This is a neocortical approach that is not acknowledging the limbic needs present. This can leave the client accurately sensing that you are not taking their pain and suffering as real.[5] I have seen people take that approach, and it simplifies people into being simply misinformed and not deeply pained by these systems.

This is not an invitation to get all the clients you see involved in the next rally, protest or political action. Indoctrinating clients into our beliefs is replicating the power structure of this society.[5] We are imposing that our idea of a better world is, in fact, better for them. There is much value in organizing as a way to increase confidence; however, your needs and their needs will never be the same. Trying to get clients to put faith in our authority instead of another is not anti-oppressive.

This is not a call to try to give clients the love they did not receive as a child. That time is over; that need is unmet. Miller is clear when she says, "The aim of therapy, however, is not to correct the past, but to enable the patient both to confront his own history and to grieve over it."[5] We can want to offer resonance and create a relational field that will hold clients as they are now, but we cannot out-love their parents into wellness. This uplifts the belief that feeling good is more important than feeling what they are actually experiencing, which is probably the same societal context that created the disconnect in the first place. This may drive clients to perform for us instead of being vulnerable.

This is not a mandate to get to work! We began this journey in Chapter 1, detailing the exhausting amount of "doing" I was in for years trying to outwork the system into liberation. This is not about focusing on being productive to fix social problems and still put aside how you experience them.[6] That is a recipe for burnout, and burnout always makes us less curious and collude instead of disrupting systems that believe individuals are not worth much if they do not produce. This is more neocortical strategy trying to meet a limbic issue.

This is not a task of becoming more informed. "In order for information to be useful to us, we have to find time to reflect on it, process it, and see if it lines up with the facts we already know."[6] Writing this book, I have been consumed with reading, writing, rereading and re-writing. I can feel I have lost my seat, I have less spaciousness, I am consumed with my own suffering, my care practices feel like distractions, I cannot meditate, my mind is always processing (more than usual) and strategizing, making me feel very resigned to its speed. This is not an anti-oppressive seat. I am ignoring my body's needs right now so I can complete this task. I am not in the place of receptivity. The more information I consume, the more I must analyze. Without the space, time and energy to reflect on new information, allowing it to impact me, it's just hoarding information, busying my mind. It does not land in my body which allows me to be impacted by the information.

This is not a sign that you need to self-improve. As a toxic culture that thrives on feeling incomplete and needing more, this would be the opposite of that. There is nothing to improve about you; there is a lot to uncover, though. Being open to surprising yourself is different than improving because it holds the stance that you don't know what you will find. It is not pushing you into a predetermined vision of the future. It's curious.

This is not an excuse to become a self-righteous, unkind person. I have been there. Getting on my pedestal and judging how mindlessly we move through living in this culture. I thought because I intellectually understood these things, I was better than others until the many times I have been knocked off my self-made pedestal by my own actions or words. You may not be able to help it; we are indoctrinated in a culture that wants us to prove our individual superiority in any shape or form, but you must pop that bubble when you notice it occurring in yourself because it will pop.

Feel Into It

What comes up in you as you read through these notes? Where is their resistance? Where is their ease?

Practice to Intervention

Are any of these impulses you usually gravitate towards? How have they looked in the past? How have clients responded? What has reinforced this strategy? What tells you you are moving in that direction? How could someone notice this in you and support you to reflect on your approach? Let your group in on what you come up with in this exploration.

Anti-Oppressive Is an Inside Job

We must accept that

> the true focus of revolutionary change is never merely the oppressive situations which we seek to escape, but that piece of the oppressor which is planted deep within each of us, and which knows only the oppressors' tactics, the oppressors' relationships.[7]

I propose that being anti-oppressive is the work of rescuing from within ourselves the seeds of nurturance, interdependence, grief and awe that have been buried under internalized oppression. This is not a linear task that we can check off; it's cyclical; it spirals, just when we think we are complete, we return. Our commitment alone is what moves us through.

Buddhist Psychology explains that in each individual person, there is a store consciousness. Within store consciousness, all the seeds of being are present. What gets watered becomes more of how we experience the world; what is unwatered lays dormant.[8] Dormant meaning, we do not utilize them because they will not help us successfully navigate our environment, so they seem non-existent. Similar to what Quantum chemists call virtual states. These states are invisible and non-existent until a molecule jumps into the state and makes it visible. Not seeing does not mean it does not exist; it just means it has not been seen yet.[9] So, the dormant seeds can be left dormant, but they can always be activated as well.

When we are used to watering the same seeds over and over again, those plants become strong, fortified and very visible, creating uninhabitable conditions for other plants to grow. The thing is, we can start watering seeds we do not see yet. What if we watered the seeds of holistic and right proportionate view rather than cognitive dissonance? What if we watered the seeds of seeing the complexity rather than categorizing? What if we watered the seeds of belonging rather than extraction? What if we watered the seeds of kinship rather than growth? What if we watered the seeds of curiosity rather than expertise? What if we watered the seeds of awe rather than knowing? What if we watered the seeds of contradictions rather than erasure?

What if we watered the seeds of is-ness rather than of illusion? What if we watered them in kinship, together? Being anti-oppressive is "not just about increasing the absence of oppression. It's also about practicing something else in its place. It's about increasing liberation."[10]

Watering the is-ness means presence. Bringing attention to the moment. Being in the is-ness often brings me right to heartbreak, hopelessness and grief. I do not plan to get over these; I do not want to heal them. As long as our collective is what it is, those emotions are the is-ness of the time and they help me navigate these times. It increases my ability to be with the heartbreak of others but also their joy.

Cultivating the Seat

"The personhood of the therapist is more central to the 'success' of the therapy than any particular technique or theoretical background."[11] Which means the attention we spend on continuing education would probably be better spent on time to reflect and engage in embodying the seat you want to occupy when you are in the counseling room. Cultivating "our personal contact with the unconscious and the irrational- these are our tools."[12] By unconscious, I mean the backstage, what has been made invisible. I have shared some general ideas on what the seat is and what it is not, but how do we cultivate an anti-oppressive seat? I have some suggestions.

Life is out of order. We need to accept that. We live in a culture that continuously wants to make life orderly, manageable, predictable and under control. That is neocortical supremacy. As we unlearn that manageable equals safety, we have space to let things be messy, unsure, and unanswered. Having a practice in surrendering control of life makes space to become curious about ourselves, the world and our connection to it. It actually makes us unafraid of being out of order. When we know we can withstand it and have harvested its fruits, our body builds an implicit memory of navigating mess.

Cultivating fearlessness of messiness and our response to messiness is powerful because it makes us receptive and relational. We can respond genuinely to those around us. Being receptive and relational is limbic; it's erotic. This erotic "becomes the lens through which we scrutinize all aspects of existence, forcing us to evaluate those aspects honestly in terms of their relative meaning with our lives."[13] That means as we get into a relationship with our erotic and limbic knowing, we begin using that to organize our world. We decrease our reliance on neocortical interpretation; instead, we feel how experiences, places and things fit within what we sense in ourselves about the world. The messiness starts to have patterns that are felt in the body, connections that are sensed. Being out of order begins to make sense.

Some reasons we do not get messy is because of our insecurities. Our insecurities are often attributes we have learned to hide or reject in response to our culture. It is where cultural narratives seep in and plant shame. Feeling towards and staying with our insecurities and shame brings us to our own complicated messiness. With the therapist shadow being strongly reliant on performing certainty- it may feel messy to not know. Being out of order is about interrupting our performance of perfectionism and confidence.[14] Where do we hide our "not knowing"? Can you go towards it and not rush it away? Getting comfortable with not knowing is a step we cannot skip.[6]

I have sat with my deep insecurity and fear of being out of order – it usually comes to me in the sense of "not knowing." When I sit with "not knowing," I feel the fear rise in me; it usually appears as confusion, nausea, heart racing and a sense that I have lost my footing and my breath. I can feel that this is young, as in it came from an implicit memory of a child version of me, but also that it is old, as in it came from my lineage. I can hear the fear in "you have to know," this voice grasping to regain control. I could never understand this sensation neocortically. I may have been able to articulate a version of it here, but the experience is in my body.

With attention and practice of returning to the sensations and emotion, I was able to see this incessant need to be knowledgeable as an overgrown plant. A plant I have been watering because I thought it was the only plant in the garden. Once I became aware that it was actually just an old plant that has been hogging all the sun and water, leaving the other plants in the shade and to be dormant, I saw the possibility for other seeds and other plants to grow. When I shift my attention away from the care of "knowing things," often I experience delight, a sense of being pleasantly surprised by the world, of being right-proportioned.

Do not get me wrong, that does not mean I do not still strive to "know things." However, now I feel limbically when I am striving to keep order. I can feel my competent stance, my "I need to know" posture, which I never noticed before because I was always in that posture. Now I get to choose if I want to keep this stance, or to soften to be vulnerable and allow myself to not know, and be open to what else is there like awe, surprise and confusion. And from that open place, everything I come in contact with feels like an experience not information to categorize and make useful.

We, as therapists who want to practice anti-oppressively, must give ourselves over to challenges that we cannot master or know our way through. We have to feel the discomfort and freedom of being out of order. Being out of order is the opposite of performing confidence. To "live in a space of transformative change is to engender greater and greater comfort with paradox."[15] Within ourselves, there are so many paradoxes; in the culture around us, there are so many paradoxes. We have to be open to conflictual realities and conflictual feelings! To not only be open, but to seek them.

Being Out of Order

Being out of order is like welcoming back all we lost to normalcy-worship.[5] So we sit with feelings we've been told are wrong, but we experience. You will learn for yourself what are some of the ways you try to control your own "messiness." Placing yourself in contradictory experiences allows your body to make new implicit memories about what can happen in the world. Sometimes, the invitation to get out of order is in hearing another experience of the world that contradicts your own. That is a great place to practice; the out-of-order feeling is nearby. With this form of attention, a curiosity may arise. You become curious about how your experience and theirs both can exist at the same time because they do. You move towards understanding how these views "become with" each other. This is not a reach across the aisle plug; it is not about being nice; this is about becoming spacious.

Being spacious in moments when we are out of order is hard, which is why we practice being with our experience when the stakes are low. Spend more time with yourself. In a culture that has a million and one ways to distract you at every given second, I know that is no easy request. "Our attention is the greatest currency of this moment – how we pay attention matters and we have to begin by paying attention to our own habituated patterns of survival."[16] Over-exertion, over-consuming information, over-scheduling ourselves to avoid discomfort will not support us in finding this seat. Spend time orienting yourself towards your own rhythms. Your body and its language. Your emotions and what they communicate about the context. Develop new tools that are not the neocortex.

Audre Lorde, in a speech to white feminists that excludes Black people, offers a well-quoted warning: "The master's tools will never dismantle the master's house."[17] To avoid this, I must understand the master's tools so I can recognize my own usage of the master's tool. To retire using those tools, I must have curiosity about my own. I need to understand the culture we are in and how it undergirds my every thought, action and impulse, including (especially) the "good" ones. I need to have enough understanding that the master's tools are, oftentimes, tools I *like* using. And learn what it feels like in me when I use them. Notice what is being rewarded with the usage of those tools, and choose whether I want to keep them or not.

There is no guidebook on which actions are or are not master's tools that I'd trust. However, with a practice of attending to myself, I can feel when I am using oppressive tools and when I am in liberation work. It can be the same action in a different context.

Let's use mindfulness as an example. For a long time, I did a mindfulness exercise every session with certain clients. Yes, there was an element of wanting to slow down and hopefully let the limbic system know it was welcomed to take more space, but it sometimes served another purpose. Sometimes, it was actually training them in how to be. Implying that calm and grounded is how you are supposed to be in therapy (remember my family execution element rant). This was essentially demonstrating to them the appropriate performance that I required from them and it also conveyed that the way they came in was wrong. For some clients, they looked forward to it because they never got the chance to slow down, and so it was a welcomed experience. For others, it was something they had to do if they wanted my help. Same action: one used as a supportive tool to inner attentiveness, and the other used to oppress and train a being, both done with sincere intention.

Now, as I have pivoted away from uniformity worship and towards practicing that there are an unimaginable number of ways to relate, I still meditate with clients, but I am paying attention to how it impacts the space between us. I check in with myself and scan if I am trying to get a need outside of my awareness met at the moment. I ask the client for guidance for when we have crossed over into performing or ritual without intention. Sometimes, I have to be honest and ask the client for a moment because *I need* to ground, and they are invited to join me, and I notice how that impacts the space between us.

And still, I do learn my own tools with meditation and mindfulness. Mindfulness is limbic because it is about the present moment. And often, there is a lot happening in my gut. Mindfulness connects the brain to the gut and heart intelligence needed for a fuller view of ourselves and where we are. "Without that heart-and gut-knowledge, we often function as 'genius-level reptiles,'" so much of what is in the gut knowledge will never be accessible through cognitive understanding, only through feeling.[18] Feeling the knowledge available in our bodies is a slow process and takes time and attention. Meditation and mindfulness allow us to slow down so that we can build the awareness needed to trust our intuition again. I think of it like we are all wandering in the dark; the neocortex is like a sharp sword cutting through hanging greenery in a rainforest to see while totally ignoring the greenery we are cutting down is the forest we are trying to see. While the limbic system starts to slowly recognize the patterns of things and the eyes begin to adjust to see in the dark. It just takes time for the eyes to learn to see where you are; you can't force it, and it shifts so slowly you may not even realize when it's changed.

Unlike how meditation is portrayed to allure the Western practitioner, it is not about feeling good or becoming a better you. It is fundamental in the movement from dissonance to resonance if you choose to engage in it in this way. Instead of thinking, strategizing, planning, debating or convincing, we can go into experiencing the ideologies we are pained by, not to fix or change, simply to not turn away from them. "It means nothing can be overlooked."[19] That means even the uncomfortable experiences that we fear will make us undone are tended to. This leads to building the skills to be out of order, present, not future-oriented or stuck in the past. Meditation is a tool of crack-staying, of sympoiesis-noticing, of limbic-remembering, of embodiment, of is-ness-being. It does not have to be sitting still meditation, although that comes with its own medicine. A practice that brings your neocortex out of planning, strategizing, categorizing and into observing the present moment will do. Being with the present moment allows for us to feel what is happening in us in response to what is happening around us. Places us back into context-connection.

Some of what can come up as we let ourselves be out of order is our personal grief. Grief "frequently waits on the other side of accepting how things are and have been."[3] An anti-oppressive therapist needs to feel this readily available pain and grief. As long as we are ignoring and hiding from it within ourselves, we will lose the fullness of a moment. As we approach grief in our bodies, our alarms may go off that we should back away; our practice teaches us when those alarms are neocortical and when they are limbic. The neocortex believes there is a world of pain we will bring on if we open that door, but what it does not know is that being with our pain is generative. It brings with it righteous rage, necessary mourning and a release that comes when we aren't working so hard to keep it together. That alone is worth it for me. The many times I have felt that relief of not needing to pretend to myself anymore. Usually, I didn't even know I was pretending at all.

Anger can make us feel out of order; however, one version makes us feel very in control. I resonate deeply with Audre Lorde when she says, "[M]y fear of anger taught me nothing. Your fear of anger will teach you nothing, also."[20] Let ourselves get angry. There is the anger I am very familiar with as a socially aware person. This anger is what lets me know "injustice is afoot," but it is the same quality of anger used to justify colonization and its horrors. The anger that comes when rights/entitlements aren't honored. In a society obsessed with having "rights," this anger can easily find the right audience to justify it. It propels me into action. It brings me out to rallies; it makes me organize; it makes me work hard. It is mostly responsible for landing me here. That anger is one that is socially accepted. We accept anger that makes us move towards getting power. That anger, although it is often hoping to use it to combat social norms, is quite neocortical and clings to concepts rather than the experience of the moment.

In New York City, the stereotype is true. It is a very common sight (you can find me doing this, too) for a pedestrian to slowly cross the street at the crosswalk even though a car is barreling down the street, with very little sign they are coming to a stop. And the pedestrian will scream, "I have the right of way!" as if that "right" will protect them from that two-and-a-half-ton piece of metal traveling at 30 miles per hour from drastically changing their lives forever in that one moment. This anger sometimes ignores reality and is foolish. Protecting rights and entitlements also brings us an anger that's harmful, that seeks a sense of dominance over other beings. This type of anger deludes us into thinking we have control over things we have no control over.[6] This anger is delusional. This anger also makes us vulnerable to collapse. When our anger is always external, we will have a million new pains to endure because we are in a culture that knows how to dish it. This anger is a recipe for losing our seat. This anger does not connect; it burns.

The anger I am speaking of here is "anger that arises over our pain and is only pointing back to our pain."[2] This anger still signals there is an "injustice afoot," yet it does not spring me into action; it grounds me in feeling the pain, hurt and grief. It brings me towards compassion, towards my precious self that must suffer. It cools me rather than heats me. This anger is the anger that brings clarity.[21] Not saying the other one does not give clarity, but it tends to lead towards projecting; this second anger brings clarity to the is-ness of the situation without looking to replicate the dominance that triggered the original pain. This anger is also shorter lasting; it rises and falls like waves. It clarifies where I am helpless; it allows me to separate that from anger that propels. It doesn't encourage strategy; it invites a falling apart, to be out of order.

The anger that clarifies might bring with it heartbreak. Let your heart break regularly. Let it feel unbearable, then let it pass until the next time. Do not waste your energy on warding off heartbreak. This does not mean "stay triggered." I have not watched, read, or engaged with the news in years. I am heartbroken enough; I do not need paralysis. When news reaches me anyway, because it does, I do not try to be strong; I let it fucking break my heart wide open. Which leads to another grief, one that is collective.

Grief and heartbreak keep the heart open and tender.[21] It is what makes us stay soft, impactable.

Grief is a path to understanding entangled shared living and dying; human beings must grieve *with*, because we are in and of this fabric of undoing. Without sustained remembrance, we cannot learn to live with ghosts and so cannot think.[22]

Mourning unsticks and makes space for movement. We don't do grief here well at all. Yet there is so much opportunity for it. There is a lot to grieve in this country, this culture and our society. So much of our cognitive dissonance energy goes towards not experiencing grief. But it is such a beautiful emotion. The more time we spend with it, the more we let it wash over us, the more we learn of its gifts. It brings rest. It comes bearing liberation. It often brings us connection if we allow it. It brings us fluidity and openness. It brings awe. Dissonance is for survival; preoccupied with an unknowable future, grief brings presence, resonates with what is living.

All of this is a conscious practice of being out of control. It is about activating our social engagement system and returning to our bodies.[23] All of these emotions are expressed by our bodies in response to the world.

"Embodiment is the work of returning home to the body, which is also to say that my awareness returns back to dwelling in my body."[2] This means we are taking back our existence, our sense of belonging to ourselves; it is not tied to or based on performance deemed pleasing by society. Trusting our bodies and the information they give is intuition. Our intuition lives in our bodies, which is different from our impulses or educated guesses. Lewis, Amini and Lannon quote a study that found that the more someone tried to think their way to solving a problem, the less their intuition could support them.[18] Intuition, like implicit memory is not summonable, but it can be felt. It can direct our actions; it can even be consulted. I know each time I feel intuition that is informed and embodied, something beautiful happens in my relational fields because "intuition brings the present moment into focus."[19] The more experiences I have with intuition, the more I trust those intuitive nudges from my gut. I perceive the world differently, not habitually. That is because "embodied transformation," by way of somatics, "is foundational change that shows in our actions, ways of being, relating and perceiving. It is transformation that sustains over time. Somatics pragmatically supports our values and actions becoming aligned"[24] Some of the changes that I have wanted to make in my life based on my values have been years of creating tricks and strategies to act differently. Yet, my body having new experiences creates lasting alignment.

Some values and actions that might arise when attending to the body are acts of caring for and seeking pleasure in our bodies again.[25] These can make you feel out of order because it is detaching from the idea of bodies as machines or hosts, and being with them as a relationship we can nurture. This is compassion. In a society that tells us that everything must be earned and everyone is competition, giving your body what it wants and needs generously and with care is a radical act. A compassionate act that creates the implicit memory of how it feels to show up generously. It is echolocation. It is believing your body, saying, "I believe you, and I will give you what you need. I want for you what you want for yourself."

Finally, what may make you feel out of order – savor your new experiences. In a culture that wants to move on to the next interesting thing, don't. Stay a while.

I thought I knew how to savor food (and not much else) until I was on silent retreat earlier this year. The food was not very good at the retreat center and, initially, I felt pain and anger of the injustice that I was being denied good food. But still, I saw that people were eating slowly, and so I imitated mindfulness because "fake it 'til you make it," amirite? But that was still a performance. As I started feeling other parts of myself that I have not been aware of rise, my experience of the meals changed. After the anger, there was a truth that my relationship with food has always been one of dissatisfaction. I had a chance to grieve how much I relied on food to escape. Then there was the pain about how hard life is that keeps me looking for escapes, seeking small moments of pleasure even if they later end with judgment or regret. I then felt the helplessness of the gravity of what was out of my control and it brought me to a very young, child-like embodiment. One where I had little control over my own suffering. She's always with me, but I could listen and attend to her because I was not consumed by avoidance. Experiencing her brought me some relief from having to work so hard at something I cannot do (control all suffering). Then there was more grief, then more relief. After a few cycles of that, I could have compassion for that little one and for myself.

Through all of this, I began enjoying the new experience of food without needing it to be anything else but nourishment for my body. Then, I had real, deeply embodied gratitude for food and how it comes to me. The spirit, land, non-human beings and the human ones, too, that allowed me to have each meal. I also held the horrors of how we do food in a colonized world, all the oppression, suffering and injustice that occurs to all those same beings I felt gratitude for. These things existed, but they were not the food itself. My desire to escape did not go away, but the food can be separate from that. When the food was detached from all of the weight I and society placed on it, it could just be food.

And I savored the hell out of that bad food. It took me almost an hour to finish a meal that would have been ten minutes tops on a regular day. I savored and sat with all this new gratitude that came with the horrors of our food industries. The savoring solidified in my system as a new experience. I could really be just tasting all that I was eating, and that felt new and exciting. It was playful. I could feel all these senses in my mouth I hadn't before. I could feel the food traveling into my stomach in a less anxious way than I ever could. It was like this very cool game of eating and noticing eating, and waiting, eating and experiencing. Have I heard of intuitive eating before? Yes. Have I read about detaching food from emotions before? Yes. Have I met people who had inspiring stories to tell? Sure. Did any of that give me the embodied feeling that would offer me new possibilities? No.

In actuality, this helped do a few things for me; although I do not eat all my meals or even most of my meals like this, I have this new sense of possibility. Like, how I am with food is not how I am, but it is how I am in a given context with food. In a different environment and context, when all my needs are being met, where I am not forced into labor for survival, when I get a chance to be with myself and have other people energetically support my experience, I can be something else, something I did now know I could be. That experience disturbed the Fundamental Attribution Error I had about myself. It reminded me that I am a collection of responses to the world around me, even when I am doing things that are seemingly "only about me," like eating.

Now, I have this additional tenderness towards other habitual escapes I am privy to in others because I am not afraid of feeling mine. I have so much tenderness that we are all figuring out this thing called life. We have developed some amazing strategies to get through this social context we are stuck in. It's all art. Each strategy. Each being. Each one. My only work as a therapist is to support someone to have space to learn what is possible for themselves. For them to see their strategies as art, not who they are.

Savoring is not an intellectual experience; it's a bodily one. We get to feel our bodies without the "holding it together" sensation. A sensation most of us do not even notice we are doing. Savoring lets us bathe in the absence of that tension and the newness of possibility that comes with just being. It is "a measure of the joy which I know myself to be capable of feeling, a reminder of my capacity for feeling."[26] This joy is different from elusive happiness or performance of happiness. This joy, delight, pleasure, play is something that only exists in this moment.

Savoring can also happen in grief and fear and other less culturally-sought emotions. Quite often, we are warding off those unsought emotions and experiences that there is a build-up, and it can be relieving to finally allow it to take over or happen. Common example is feeling as though you have had a big cry building up for weeks. Finally, something small happens and triggers this big cry. The idea of crying may have been off-putting, and so it was avoided, but the cry itself feels good. That is something to savor. Savoring is very aware that every moment is a unique moment that has never happened before and will never happen again – so soak it in.

Wrapping Up

Unfortunately, most of us do not get to stop working for a while to get out of control, feel all our feelings, be in our bodies and then return to work as limbically attuned and caring therapists. And this is a location of practice in itself. To be with our livelihood being connected to our ability to work. Wrestle with how we are perceived as good for doing this work. Struggle with the truth that although we have not perfected life, we are still sought out as an expert on it. Confront the disconnect between the theories that we utilize in our practices and how we actually live. Take on wanting to heal our past experiences or rectify an imagined future through clients. Toss and turn about how we sustain this sociopathic culture. Becoming undone is not a one-time event. It is a practice. Just keep reminding yourself: the goal is not to fix – that's delusional – the goal is to be with.

Feel Into It

Feel into the Seat. How does it feel here? What thoughts is your mind clinging to? What makes you feel far away from the seat? What makes you feel close?

You can discuss why that is with your group – for now just notice and express.

Citations

1. Hassan, S. (2022). *Saving our own lives: A liberatory practice of harm reduction* (D. G. Lewis, Ed.). Haymarket Books.
2. Owens, L. R. (2020). *Love and rage: The path of liberation through anger.* North Atlantic Books.
3. Feinberg, B. (2018). Undiscovering the Pueblo Mágico: Lessons from Huautla for the psychedelic renaissance. *Plant Medicines, Healing and Psychedelic Science*, 37–54. https://doi.org/10.1007/978-3-319-76720-8_3
4. Maté, G., MD, & Maté, D. (2022). *The myth of normal: Trauma, illness, and healing in a toxic culture.* Avery.
5. Miller, A. (1997). *The drama of the gifted child: The search for the true self* (revised ed., 3rd ed.). Basic Books.
6. Price, D., PhD. (2022). *Laziness does not exist.* Atria.
7. Lorde, A. (2007). Age, race, class and sex: Women redefining difference. In *Sister outsider*. The Crossing Press. (Original work published 1983)
8. Hanh, N. T. (2023). *Understanding our mind by Nhat Hanh, Thich [Paperback].* Parallax, 2006.
9. Ponte, D., & Schäfer, L. (2013). Carl Gustav Jung, quantum physics and the spiritual mind: A mystical vision of the twenty-first century. *Behavioral Sciences*, 3(4), 601–618. https://doi.org/10.3390/bs3040601
10. Birdsong, M. (2020). *How we show up: Reclaiming family, friendship, and community.* Hachette Go.
11. Murphy, J. (2015). The therapeutic relationship in Hakomi therapy. In H. Weiss, L. Monda, & G. Johanson (Eds.), *Hakomi mindfulness-centered somatic psychotherapy: A comprehensive guide to theory and practice* (1st ed.). W.W. Norton & Company, Inc.
12. Guggenbühl-Craig, A. (1996). *Power in the helping professions* (12th ed.). Spring Publications, Inc.
13. Lorde, A. (2019). Uses of the erotic: The erotic as power. In A. M. Brown (Ed.), *Pleasure activism: The politics of feeling good.* AK Press. (Original work published 1984)
14. Harrison, D. L., & Laymon, K. (2021). *Belly of the beast: The politics of anti-fatness as anti-blackness.* North Atlantic Books.
15. Williams, A. K., Owens, R., & Syedullah, J., PhD. (2016). *Radical dharma: Talking race, love, and liberation* (Illustrated). North Atlantic Books.
16. Leiner, R., & Syedullah, J. (2023). The manual for liberating survival: Lesson I, how self-care matters as an embodied practice of abolition. In A. Crawley & R. Sirvent (Eds.), *Spirituality and abolition.* Common Notions.
17. Lorde, A. (2007). The master's tools will never dismantle the master's house. In *Sister outsider*. Ten Speed Press.

18. Lewis, T., Amini, F., & Lannon, R. (2001). *A general theory of love* (Reprint). Vintage.

19. Stanley, J. (2021). *Yoke: My yoga of self-acceptance*. Workman Publishing Company.

20. Lorde, A. (2007). The uses of anger: Women responding to racism. In *Sister outsider*. The Crossing Press. (Original work published 1983)

21. Thanissara. (2015). *Time to stand up: An engaged Buddhist manifesto for our earth -- The Buddha's life and message through feminine eyes (sacred activism)* (1st ed.). North Atlantic Books.

22. Haraway, D. J. (2016). *Staying with the trouble: Making Kin in the Chthulucene (experimental futures)* (Illustrated). Duke University Press Books.

23. Morgan, M. (2015). The central role of the body in Hakomi psychotherapy. In H. Weiss, L. Monda, & G. Johanson (Eds.), *Hakomi mindfulness-centered somatic psychotherapy: A comprehensive guide to theory and practice* (1st ed.). W.W. Norton & Company, Inc.

24. Brown, A. M. (2019). Feeling from within. In *Pleasure activism: The politics of feeling good*. AK Press.

25. Taylor, S. R. (2018). *The body is not an apology: The power of radical self-love* (16pt large print ed.) (Large type/Large print). ReadHowYouWant.

26. Lorde, A. (2019). Uses of the erotic: The erotic as power. In A. M. Brown (Ed.), *Pleasure activism: The politics of feeling good*. AK Press. (Original work published 1984)

Part 3

Practice Limbic Resonance

Chapter 8

Shaping Cultural Evolution

So, in the last chapter, we felt into all these emotions, but remember, limbic systems are not individual; they need others. "In order to be utilized," feelings "must be recognized. The need for sharing deep feeling is a human need."[1] We are not only our inner worlds; we are our relationships. Donna Haraway pushes the slogan "Make Kin Not Babies" because we are steadily overpopulating the planet.[2] Overpopulation is a major contributor to the Anthropocene. In this culture, it is easier to create a new life that is dependent on receiving your care than working to be in intimate relationships, dependent relationships, vulnerable relationships. Our individuation makes this feel normal, but it is actually cognitive dissonance that ignores our longing for interdependence. Because there is an "interconnected intimacy that is messy, uncomfortable, and difficult, but worthy and liberating to attend to."[3]

In societies that are truly autonomous but not individual, they only care for their connected kin, like the Matsigenka of the Peruvian Amazon.[4] Henrich learned from the Matsigenka people when visiting that they have no interest in scaling up, no interest in being part of something bigger; they live with their connected kin and stay away from those who interrupt their peace. They reside and live in small kin groups far away from each other. I see this as a beautiful blueprint for liberation. Engaged in smaller, truly autonomous and nurturing connections that are committed to each other. In our context, time and place, our groups may not be genetically related. Well, relatives in the early English language meant "logical relations" not family members.[2] However, we have deprioritizing logic up to this point. So, let's embody a new approach to relatives, relations that are limbic and resonant.

Relatives: The Kin That Holds the Practitioner

For the shadow side of the healer/doctor to survive, it needs to be isolated, it needs to be superior and it cannot tolerate challenges to that. So, to occupy the anti-oppressive seat, we must be in groups where we are challenged. Where we are held accountable. We should take in critiques with care and study them.[5] We

DOI: 10.4324/9781003207054-11

must have plenty of opportunities to be directed towards being out of control so we can see for ourselves what lurks there. To create a nurturance culture, accountability is necessary.[6] Nurturance culture is the opposite of rape culture, which is one of dominance over others. I consider nurturance culture one that is limbically attuned and steeped in sympoietic relationships. In these relationships, we must believe about ourselves and each other this: "[W]e are not our worst behaviors."[7] This increases our willingness to handle rupture and expect repair.

Pods, a Transformative Justice foundation given this name and form by Mia Mingus and Bay Area Transformative Justice Collective, are a limbic strategy. They "are made up of the people in our lives we turn to first and rely on."[8] Because in a society that builds community based on identity or market value, community continues to be elusive. Many people feel as though they do not have or have never had one. Pods are intentional and consented to and probably already exist in your life. It isn't about building new relationships; it is about leaning into trusting relationships. The accountability necessary for the psychotherapist rests on the established trust of their relationships and the collective practices they have developed. Practicing accountability disrupts the dispositionalism-based falsity that "only bad people do bad things."[8] Believing we are not our worst behavior and having established trusting relationships creates the conditions to accept that context matters. Accepting that hurt and harm happens, this condition fuels the commitment to address, repair and heal from hurt and keeps those hurts from becoming part of shadow.

Kinship-based cultures do not need to create explicit accountability pods; they are ingrained into accountability to the group norms. Due to the size of our society, accountability is not based on group cohesion, it is based on universalism and used for control and often conflated with the word and concert of punishment. In smaller, intimate groups there can be accountability that is responsive to context and is relational. Accountability is not only a response to when something bad happens. The other side is gratitude, recognizing when a person is showing up well in a relationship. Both are about allowing yourself to be seen and reflected. They allow others to share how your being plays with/impacts/resonates with their being. It's a practice in "becoming with." Whether you call it pods, community, kin – we need it. As a clinician, your only form of accountability cannot be your client. First, because there is a power differential, no matter how much you would like to strike it down, and secondly, because they do not see enough of you. We need accountability from friends, family, supervisors and colleagues. People who see more of us, different parts of us.

Here, I will share some wise guidance from Malidoma Patrice Somé. Community is based on consent from community members that acknowledge "the possibility of doing together what is impossible to do alone."[9] He goes on to share that a community does not need a police force; if it has one, that means the community is not working. A community cannot be based on opposing another community. So, having a community that only wants to be *anti*-oppressive cannot survive. Having shared language and political leanings will not sustain the relationships and trust needed to maintain this quality of community. This is still very neocortically built. Ego-mate driven. It is not responsive to the community members; it's responsive to concepts external to them. A community "is not a place where you reform, but a place you go home to,"[9] meaning the kin-group is supporting each other as is. This does not mean they will not offer feedback and have accountability measures, but it means they trust one another to be with what is showing up. This is a sympoietic practice. It devalues good, bad, right or wrong and tolerates complexity. It accepts the impact of the moment and chooses how to respond. This is echolocation. Like, "Ok, this happened, we are here now. Let's not shut down. Let's feel what this makes us now. How do we metabolize this?"

As well as being accountable, the practitioner also needs to be liberated from isolation. We need connection. Connection that allows us to transform narcissistic lover energy to mature nurturer. Thanissara explains that a mature nurturer is not consumed with personal love and attention but stands with fierce love that protects and defends.[10] In Western culture, friendships are meant to protect autonomy and sustain individualism, which often preserves delusions.[11] It also means friends are using each other, oftentimes without knowing. Audre Lorde warns, "[W]hen we look away from ourselves as we satisfy our erotic needs in concert with others, we use each other as objects of satisfaction rather than share our joy in the satisfying."[1] That kind of connection is neocortical. It is about keeping our performance together, not about putting them aside and being embodied together, resonating.

We can borrow some philosophy from adrienne maree brown, who describes liberated relationships as the remedy to using each other. Brown shares a three-pronged model for liberated relationships. They consist of radical honesty, they acknowledge dynamics such as social/cultural/emotional contexts that affect the relationship and they relinquish the desire to fix or make the other in the relationship different.[12] Mia Birdsong adds another dimension to consider when making friends – that these relationships aspire to real freedom. "Freedom was the idea that together we can ensure that we all have the things we need – love, food, shelter, safety."[13] So they are also invested in your literal livelihood, and you in theirs.

Radical honesty requires trust. Acknowledging dynamics requires mutual study. Relinquishing the desire to fix means accepting. Investing in each other requires vulnerability. These qualities of relationships are not about collecting people around you. These relationships need time, lots of attention and intention to create the conditions necessary so they can unfold.[14] In a society that moves urgently and is quick to dispose of everything, this is a courageous and risky business.

For this to work, we must resist the norm of disposing of people. In our culture, because we aren't kin-tied, we make relationships that need to produce, and if someone isn't producing the right experience, feeling, aesthetic then we are encouraged to leave them and find other people. That's disposability. People not doing things to our liking does not make them disposable if we are committed to being in a kin-inspired relationship. This is not an invitation to invite any ole body into your life; this is for your connections, not your community (in this culture, we say community, and that can mean a couple of million people). We have to consciously and effortfully do the opposite of throwing away.

> [W]e need to flood the entire system with life-affirming principles and practices, to clear the channels between us of the toxicity of supremacy, to heal from the harms of a legacy of devaluing some lives and needs in order to indulge others.[15]

By choosing to stay and not dispose, we are creating new collective experiences of being valuable just as you are, not because of what you produce.

These connections must hold spirit. This does not mean an organized religion. This means that when you are present and spirit moves you, the group can honor that in you. That these connections engage in the ritual that arises out of the moment. Malidoma Patrice Somé speaks and writes a lot about the great depravity of the West is the loss of ritual.[9] We need ritual to connect us to land, body, spirit and each other. We also need rituals to mark a moment in time. These care connections must make space for all the unknown that is amongst you already. This is not an invitation to find a ritual online and to replicate it, although you may be inspired by one. Investigate your history and lineage with ritual. Grieve that. Keep grieving. Respectfully observe or contribute to the rituals of others, speak to ritual holders. Feel what they spring up in you or make available to you, and then dream. Dream about what you need in your ritual in this context, this place and this time.

Ritual and spirituality are adaptive, always responding to the land, place in time, spirit, organism and the need of organisms. Ritual is sympoietic. That means a group's rituals must reflect the group. It is not a one-size-fits-all world. Where the group is located, the dynamics within the group, the values of the group and their practices in resonating together will make every ritual different. Spirit work is about reclaiming kinship. "Animism cannot be donned like a magic cape."[2] Animism is knowing that all things have life and must be interacted with as such. There needs to be an effort to build these relationships with non-human beings, too. These relationships can teach the rituals the group needs.

All of these types of relationships are hard-won in this culture. And honestly, we are not equipped to be in these types of relationships because of the elements that have shaped us. They require lots of time, effort, vulnerability, intimacy, unlearning, mistakes, ruptures and slowness. Thankfully, our limbic system is up for the task. In other cultures, this is a truly foreign concept – searching for and longing for loving relationships. In many cultures, you do not examine who gets or does not get your care. "You have to take care of the people with whom you are dependent."[11] That kinship is not value-based; it's dependency-based.

If we accept that our nation is our family, a concept created to scale up, dependency-based kinship is impossible. But if we were to practice being sympoietic, partners in becoming with the land we actually occupy, the critters we are exposed to, the people we spend time with, support, who support us, who hold us accountable to our values, who make space for the slow limbic unfurling, then we can do kinship. Kinship that accepts that emotions are between us and the embodied expressions of them gives us permission to stop performing. They remind us we matter without it being about entitlements. This quality of kinship is radical. When we progressives imagine the future we are fighting for and all we can dream up are large-scale systems and structural changes, we are setting ourselves up for a future that will never come. Kat shares simply that "there is no utopia but our relationships. A sustainable revolution must value existing relationships instead of attempting to make the world anew. A sustainable revolution must learn to live with the world we have."[16] That means instead of waiting for the perfect people, perfect conditions, try small movements towards the relationships you can be more vulnerable with, now.

Feel Into It

Create a pod map. Go to www.soiltjp.org/our-work/resources/pods to learn more. Share your pod map with your group. Then, share your pod map with those you have included in it.

What does it feel like in your body to be given this assignment? What do you know about these embodied emotional experiences?

The Self That Does Kin

Caring for ourselves and our bodies is a vital part of liberation. To be in these qualities of relationships, we need capacity, spaciousness, attention to give, care to offer. When we are overworked, stressed, tired, malnourished, burned out, dazed by existential dread, disconnected from our bodies- we have nothing to give. We cannot be responsive to others. We cannot show up when others need us. Taking care of ourselves is part of being in community. "It's about learning the limits of your capacity" rather than blowing past our capacity and having nothing left to be relational with those we love.[17] It's about experiencing compassion, so we have it to give to others. It is about reorienting away from the patterns we have adapted to survive our conditions and towards cultivating the conditions we want to become in. Unlike Chapter 7, where we cultivate awareness on our own, we can also cultivate awareness with others.

I would recommend having a therapist, healer and some practitioners as kin. Listen, I love me a good healer, divinator and practitioner of spiritual arts, but in our society, so much is wrapped in ideas we have of ourselves and the world. Ideally, talk therapy is where those can be revealed and worked with in slow form. Therapists must be the first ones in their own therapy. Find someone who will direct you back to your own body for the information you seek, who will move at the speed of resonance, not strategy. Take your time; find the people who will support you in the reunification of your backstage and performance. Having this space is vital to learning how it feels to embody a relational field that is nurtured and attended to. Often, it is our first real understanding of what is possible through limbic connection.

Get stellar supervision. Have someone or a group dedicated to showing you yourself and how you are showing up in the power seat. Professional or Work pods are a thing.[8] People committed to showing you when cognitive dissonance has you ignoring certain complicated pieces of information in yourself, others and moments. When you are colluding with social values of being good, healthy, normal and productive. When you are only attending to one element or lens. When you are using your neocortex to solve a limbic issue that does not need solving. We need people to shake us up, help us find the messiness to occupy for a while. Remember, we are abandoning our profession – so push away from what a "professional setting" or "professional community" is supposed to look like. Expect and encourage the vulnerable. Seek the limbic. Make the invisible visible. Make it uncomfortable.

Call on the unseen for support. That can look many ways. It takes time, commitment, guidance, trial and error to find the unseen that draws you. The unseen can be microscopic, like the M. paradoxa, or be natural elements like wind, water, earth, fire, etc. It can be the spirits of the living world. Ancestors in your biological lineage or another that has drawn you. This disrupts our anthropogenic tendencies towards self-centeredness and puts us in right-proportion. It knocks us down from our superiority, not making anything else more superior but recognizing there is more at play in our lives than our will alone. This seeks to make kin with more than human beings. To invite mystery and unknowns. To be receptive. To water our dormant seeds.

Feel Into It to Find It

I hope what is abundantly clear is that you cannot dismantle isolation in isolation. You cannot dismantle dominance with dominance. You cannot dismantle neocortex supremacy with your neocortex. This anti-oppressive/liberatory seat isn't somewhere I can instruct you on how to find. You feel it. And you keep feeling it until you find it. Then you lose it and feel into it to find it again. The seat is about learning to care for ourselves rather than our performances or a society that is never satiated.[9]

All of this practice, invoking the erotic through exploring being out of order; experiencing the emotions and truths we push away like grief, anger and compassion; allowing their medicines to surface like relief, delight, pleasure and joy; feeling all this in your body; sharing these experiences with kin; allowing those kin to be intimately in your becoming and you in theirs; finding kinship in non-human beings; all of this practice is about creating new implicit memory. It is about replacing explicit directives to be productive and useful. Like the implicit braider mentioned in Chapter 4, we do not need to know *how* to do it to do it. This connection to others allows us to pull away from the violence of the state to have our needs met.[7] It brings our loyalty to each other, our kin. I strongly believe this is how we impact Cultural Evolution; this is our contribution to the collective consciousness.

There are examples of this in physics. The term nonlocality means "when two particles which at one time interact and then move away from one another, can stay connected and act as though they were one thing, no matter how far apart they are."[18] I interpret this to mean if we are creating our small intimate kin-groups, we are moving as one; we are sympoietic; we are shifting our collective. Zapatista Pablo Gonzalez Casanova shared a sign for progressive movements: "[T]he project will have succeeded when the struggles for autonomy have evolved into networks of autonomous peoples."[19]

Our kin-groups will shape our world. This usage of the language "shape" comes from the parable series written by Octavia E. Butler, who inspired many of my teachers. In the series, a common chorus is "God is change."[20] Furthermore, the heroine uplifts that we can shape change and, therefore, shape God. In this spirit, kin-groups are not dormant, self-indulgent, static organisms; they can move; they create; they shape change. If one pod member has experienced a harm, that means the pod shows up. And the individuals in the pod have pods that show up for them. And so forth. This is different from scaling up; this is mycelial. Adrienne maree brown brought this concept into my consciousness. Mycelium is a network of fungus roots below the ground; it "is the largest organism on earth."[21] It is not dormant; it acts. Movement work isn't only the aggressive, power-shifting kind, it is also the ground-shifting kind. This is actually how cultural evolution happens. This can be building the models for what happens after the world economy is no longer viable. It will be too late then to try to learn how to show up for each other.

Feel free to borrow my anchor when I become anxious and urgent about the speed of change, which is a quote by Dr. Jasmine Syedullah: "It is not enough to know we want freedom. We have to practice it."[21] It reminds me that this moment is a moment to practice. I can check in, "How are my relations?" Relations to my body, mind, spirit, kin, land, non-human beings, the unseen and other. What connections can I melt into right now that remind me of the freedom of this moment? Bringing me back into the limbic present, drawing me out of the cultural isolation strategy, reminding me that the freedom I seek is here.

Citations

1. Lorde, A. (2019). Uses of the erotic: The erotic as power. In A. M. Brown (Ed.), *Pleasure activism: The politics of feeling good*. AK Press. (Original work published 1984)
2. Haraway, D. J. (2016). *Staying with the trouble: Making Kin in the Chthulucene (experimental futures)* (Illustrated). Duke University Press Books.
3. Manuel, Z. E. (2015). *The way of tenderness: Awakening through race, sexuality, and gender*. Wisdom Publications.
4. Henrich, J. (2021). *WEIRDest people in the world: How the west became psychologically peculiar and particularly prosperous*. Picador Paper.
5. Guggenbühl-Craig, A. (1996). *Power in the helping professions* (12th ed.). Spring Publications, Inc.
6. Samaran, N. (2019). *Turn this world inside out: The emergence of nurturance culture*. AK Press.
7. Hassan, S. (2022). *Saving our own lives: A liberatory practice of harm reduction* (D. G. Lewis, Ed.). Haymarket Books.
8. Mingus, M. (2023, March 16). *SOILTJP – PODS*. www.soiltjp.org/our-work/resources/pods
9. Somé, M. P. (1997). *Ritual: Power, healing and community (compass)* (1st ed.). Penguin Books.
10. Thanissara. (2015). *Time to stand up: An engaged Buddhist manifesto for our earth -- The Buddha's life and message through feminine eyes (sacred activism)* (1st ed.). North Atlantic Books.
11. Mesquita, B. (2022). *Between us: How cultures create emotions*. W. W. Norton & Company.
12. Brown, A. M. (2019). *Pleasure activism: The politics of feeling good*. AK Press.
13. Birdsong, M. (2020). *How we show up: Reclaiming family, friendship, and community*. Hachette Go.
14. Woodland, E., & Page, C. (2023). *Healing justice lineages: Dreaming at the crossroads of liberation, collective care, and safety*. North Atlantic Books.
15. Brown, A. M., & Devich-Cyril, M. (2020). *We will not cancel us: And other dreams of transformative justice (Emergent Strategy Series, 3)*. AK Press.
16. Kat, S. A. (2021). *Postcolonial astrology: Reading the planets through capital, power, and labor*. North Atlantic Books.
17. Leiner, R., & Syedullah, J. (2023). The manual for liberating survival: Lesson I, how self-care matters as an embodied practice of abolition. In A. Crawley & R. Sirvent (Eds.), *Spirituality and abolition*. Common Notions.
18. Ponte, D., & Schäfer, L. (2013). Carl Gustav Jung, quantum physics and the spiritual mind: A mystical vision of the twenty-first century. *Behavioral Sciences, 3*(4), 601–618. https://doi.org/10.3390/bs3040601
19. Rojas, P. X. (2017). Are the cops in our heads and hearts? In INCITE! (Ed.), *The revolution will not be funded: Beyond the non-profit industrial complex*. Duke University. (Original work published 2006)
20. Butler, O. E. (2014). *Parable of the sower*. Hachette UK.
21. Williams, A. K., Owens, R., & Syedullah, J., PhD. (2016). *Radical dharma: Talking race, love, and liberation* (Illustrated). North Atlantic Books.

Chapter 9

Colluding with Liberation

Feel into It

Breathe here. We are coming to the end. Feel your body, this body, the body you have right now. As it is. Sense into this moment wherever you are, whatever time it is, whoever you are with, how your body is responding to all of it. Let yourself rest here for a bit before proceeding.

Practice to Intervention

How have these Feel Into It prompts changed for you? Or haven't? Go back and reflect on the first few prompts. How did you engage with those? How about now? What's changed? What can you take from this exploration about you?

So, how do you use the last eight chapters in working with clients?

I must end with apologies, just as I began. This chapter will disappoint. I am sorry this is not a "how to" guide; this is a "feel through" invitation. Because if I have not expressed it enough, your own system, the context you are in, the world of the client and collective history present are what will inspire your next move. This book cannot capture the combinations you will find yourself in. But I have some general advice that you can sense your way through towards having a liberatory practice for the people you serve.

Engaging with the Other Seat

The anti-oppressive practice requires us to be deeply intimate with contradictions. For example, I have my analysis about how pride brings along a shadow of shame in this culture; I have done all this personal work unlearning around this unnatural connection between the two and in myself; and I have sat with shame

DOI: 10.4324/9781003207054-12

and felt the relief of experiencing it rather than guarding against it; I speak to my kin about it and we all feel held in our vulnerability and have had beautiful corrective experiences. This experience of mine cannot be forced onto a client. I cannot go into a session where someone wants to experience personal pride and say, "Maybe try shame instead. You know our society blah blah blah." This is neocortex to neocortex working. I can, however, sit squarely and spaciously in my seat with an engaged and receptive limbic system that is tracking myself and us. From there, I can accept that we will be working towards experiencing pride because there is no right way of doing anything, and I am following the lead of the client. If the loudest voice in the room is wanting pride, I am going to go with it. If there is another voice that may not be verbal that holds the shame, I am going to track it and name it, and let it become visible. Then, I may lead us to look at it. But I cannot guess it is there because I intellectually link the two. I need to feel its presence between us. Sometimes, it's an experience of it in myself that tells me. A sensation that I, too, am hiding from shame or working to keep it away. Sometimes, it's the gestures in the other person or assumptions I hear in their content.

However, for so many of us, the neocortex is so steeped in the world, and it has always been the loudest voice in the room; I must accept that, too. That sometimes there is only what is being said. What I do in those situations, I hold a wish in myself; at some point, I do say it out loud when we've visited enough, and I have the intuition that they may have that wish, too. But I hold this wish limbically because if I hold it neocortically, it will drive me to do something/ impose something; I want it to be passive and present. This wish is always aligned with wanting their limbic system to start taking up more space. And one day, that desire for feeling pride will be right-proportioned and make space for something else. Something else not known to me or the client yet. This is the level of contradiction I'm talking about.

If it takes all this cycling of unraveling, feeling pain, anger, grief, heartbreak and savor in becoming undone of Chapter 7 to find our seat, imagine what then does it take for the person in the seat opposite us. That is where we want to approach that seat from. What does it take to be you? How is your way of navigating your world a reflection of my world? How can my ongoing deconstruction of my world make me a soft landing spot for you? How can my vulnerability and access to me create a relational field primed to limbically resonate with you? What feels within the realm of possibility for you? What seems in the realm of impossibility for me? How can I feel your being as one intertwined with mine? Where am I tangled up in your story? Where am I far away?

Ritual

All of this being with ourselves and in connection is so that we can feel into the generative possibilities of embodiment. If we have experienced it enough, we learn to look for how to bring it. We become open to whatever arises because we trust our bodies, intuition and our relationships to support us in metaboliz-ing new information, even hard information. This actually allows us to move into unknowns with a state of "willingness instead of willfulness."[1] Willing to be with what happens, not willful to make things happen. This way of being is called Loving Presence in Hakomi, the therapist's greatest tool. Loving presence is what I feel when I read Lama Rod Owens write about his practice: "It helps me remain present to what others are feeling because I am present to my own situa-tion."[2] When we are attending to this between us, we are caring for the relational field. The relational field is the space between our limbic system and another's. Whether it is attuned to or not, it is present. It is influencing the space. In it are a lot of said and unsaid, felt and unfelt things. We tend to the relational field so we can make visible the invisible between us (recall virtual states).

The relational field is not candles, plants and soft colors on the wall. All of that will invite the neocortex in, but the limbic system is geared towards what actually happens between those pastel-colored walls or in front of our well-manicured Zoom background. The relational field is not about making it pleas-ant; it's about cultivating a container you can both vulnerably step into.

Attending to the relational field is a ritual. Rituals have clearly marked begin-nings, middles and ends. Rituals must have purpose. Engaging the relational field is an invitation to the limbic systems in the space saying, "I am ready to experience you as you are." That is the purpose of this type of ritual. Like many rituals, it is to mark utilizing other than regular consciousness. It is to bring forth the unseen, the unsaid, the unfelt and to trust that through this ritual, new infor-mation and possibilities can arise. Rituals need to be closed. We must invite the clients back into their regular consciousness and bring the neocortex back into the space. We do not leave our client open and abandon them in the unknown; that is an unclosed ritual. It is important to re-invite the neocortex that makes sense of our limbic experiences (as much as it can). The neocortex makes the experiences into places we can choose to visit or conjure whenever we want, not only in ritual space.

Treat the ritual like a visit. Haraway describes Hannah Arendt's words "to go visiting"[3] as meaning to, almost fully, suspend all you know so you can have sin-cere curiosity about the world you are visiting together or the world of another. It includes doing "the energetic work of holding open possibility that surprises are in store, that something *interesting* is about to happen, but only if one cultivates the virtue of letting those one visits intra-actively shape what occurs."[3] In other words, there is no new information when you try to maintain control or cling to what you know.

We visit with humility.

Moving with humility means we honor the space between what we know, what we do not yet know, and what is unknowable. It requires decentering ourselves and our ego to be open to learning, regardless of years of training and so-called expertise.[4]

I like thinking of sessions as ritual because it defies dominance, it goes against forward motion; it pauses; it begins; it ends; it can never be duplicated because it's responsive to the moment, even if the actions are repeated, it will never be the same ritual twice.[5] Whatever happens between opening and closing must come from the "pit of your belly," as Dagara village members would say.[5]

But the pit of our belly is often actually in our heads in this culture, and its pit is dominance, analytic supremacy and colonization. We must be careful when entering another's world because "we have been educated to do something, and as therapists we are tempted to force things 'for the client's own good.'"[6] Being allowed in someone's world is deeply honorable yet can pull at our training and dispositions towards being useful. To combat this, we must remember ritual is about being willing, not willful. It is about utilizing your real pit, in your belly, the limbic knowing. To do this, you must practice distinguishing where intuition comes from.

My friend and colleague Angella Okawa shares the wisdom of Maria Lugones, who offers guidance on how to avoid the pitfalls of "making things happen." She builds this image of traveling through worlds without conquering them. This is hard since, in our culture, traveling is often in an attempt to conquer another. Angella shares that this may happen when someone unintentionally imposes "their understanding of their world onto another world, thus 'killing' it."[7] Not only are we killing the world of the other, but we are killing any possibility for unknown worlds to appear. Lugones offers playfulness as a wise way to travel worlds without conquering them. This playfulness includes being open to surprise, open to seeming foolish, open to reconstruction of self and open to reconstruction or construction of the world you share.[7]

When we aren't taking ourselves so seriously, we can listen so deeply "that we are open to being changed."[7] What comes out of these types of rituals are new possibilities that meet the reality of the moment. But the moment must be fully felt and experienced; that is the ritual.

Feel Into It

Ritual. What is conjured in you as we go through the possibilities of session as ritual?

Practice to Intervention

I am not sure what to do about virtual therapy. I am saddened by it and concerned about its limitations and influence on the field. I can, of course, feel how much of myself is relaxed when I am in my home, only seen from the chest up, but I also can feel how much is absent by not having that connection. Although I can still sense our relational field, it requires more words, more effort to engage in. It was so different when we were able to breathe each other in. The relational field is severely compromised when virtual – because a computer has no limbic sense. I must be honest that I am continuing to do Zoom because it's convenient for me and the people I serve. Thankfully, I do see most of them in person at times, but not enough. I am continuing to figure out this new place we've found ourselves in. But I want to be clear that we must hold onto what is missed when we are fully virtual. I think there is a lot to come in my practice around this crack.

What can ritual look like in a growing virtual field? With shorter sessions? And more prescriptive ideas of success in therapy? These are what I grapple with these days. What do you think?

Tending to the Relational Field

To be fully curious about their world, you have to have a good understanding that "the world" is made up. You have to know that "your" world is not "the" world, that it's a bunch of projections. To enter that space, you cannot have energy going into the maintenance of your backstage. There must be an acceptance that some things that tend to be pushed backstage may be aroused when in the company of other beings. Through your own work, you will be able to stay present and tend to yourself because it is all part of the field. Accepting that and having practices set up will allow you to be pulled into your client's world. Allowing their world to open up and initiate you in its ways. Not their thoughts or analysis about their world, but what it feels like to be a member of their world. The relational field allows for sensations that may never have words to be communicated. And when you encounter them, you shouldn't bother trying to understand; you can just feel it, too, and it will instruct you on what comes next.

Let us be careful here. Although we are creating a relational field and will actively and willingly engage in limbic resonance, we are not correcting experiences for our clients. What happened, happened. We are also not modeling other relationships with them because emotions change based on relationships.[8] What happens with us will not happen with their loved ones. This belief that we are fine substitutes for loved ones is the Fundamental Attribution Error in action. It relies on the belief that we are the same no matter the context. And also true, but in contradiction, that through implicit memory, clients are learning a new possibility of being with us.[9] They can activate how they get to show up with us in other areas of their lives that will give them a road map of how they want to feel in that different context.

The relational field also does not mean always being nice. It means being open; it means being accepting and vulnerable, and to do that, we cannot collude with deception. The anti-oppressive clinician disrupts deception by speaking to it.[10] We do not collude with the deception of norms. There will be many times when a client is between a norm that seems to be the right answer and a more difficult truth being avoided. It is the honor of the therapist to bear witness and point out that it seems that the rules of the norm must be broken here[11] and let our client see this other option.

Until you get the hang of the speed of your own system, move slowly. Slow yourself down. Slow the client down. It's ok to take a long time to respond and see what shifts in the relational field. Everything, intentional or not, is information in the field. Do not be fragile, and try to control what is in the field. This does not mean use the field to poke at the client; it means seeing them as precious, but the field is not. You can do this when you've had enough experience in your system of not being disposed of, repair and reconciliation.

Be transparent. Say what you are considering out loud. It is already in the field. I see a client who, every time I start trying to put some things together, she says, "I see you are about to do that Florie thing," and she is almost always right. I was about to make some connections. I do not want to replicate powerful, impenetrable, sage demi-gods. I want to be human, and that means not playing the role of "ole wise one," that everything must come out as a stroke of genius. If you are following something in your system or in theirs, name it. You are a tool for their liberation, not the master of it.

We must let the clients know we know some things, but the expert in the room is always them. That we heed to the expertise in the room. We release our agendas and our treatment plans. We let our system work for theirs like an informant. When we notice something, we toss it back in the field for them to make sense of it with our total attention.

This Is a Practice

My friend, colleague and sometimes muse Tayla Shanaye writes, "[B]e it finding times for stillness, surrendering to play, or releasing a wash of tears, I'm reminded about the essential practice of *presence*."[12]

Practice of presence is an experimental attitude. We need an experimental attitude. Not like in scientific research, where we are looking to prove our hypothesis correct. Child-like play, like tasting mud, because it's there, and we aren't sure what to make of it. Our curiosity and the attunement will tell us what to drop in the field or allow us to see what is already brewing. That will change moment to moment. People are not stagnant beings. Our worlds can shift at any moment. We must hold so preciously whatever we perceive of the clients today, let it pass through us without attachment and then next week be ready to start again and meet a new world. Ready to be re-invited into their world, ready to know more. We can do it with them because we practice it with ourselves first.

It is a practice because we will never perfect any of this; we get to be constant learners.

The Invitation

All of what I shared in this chapter are lifetime practices. I am no expert, since I am still living. It took you your whole life, plus the lives of generations before you; it took us 200,000 years of cultural evolution to get to where we are now. We cannot expect to have a different world tomorrow, but we can expect that we actually are not sure what tomorrow will be and meet it with curiosity and a sense of possibility.

Notice that nowhere in here do I say, then start building a big practice, or start small and get big. Scaling up is the monster that continues to rob us of the connections our human systems are designed for. Nothing needs to be for everyone. I understand in capitalism, it's hard not to see scaling up as the way to free yourself. But with all you know now, let the discomfort of the paradox come, too. If you are working in a clinic, let the contradictions be there. If you are running a private practice, let the sacrifices disturb you. If you weren't willing, I do not think you would be reading this (unless you were forced to; in that case, you do you). So let whatever brought you here keep you in the tension and never let you reside fully in dissonance again. The great pain is and has been disconnection, and to reconnect, we do not need more dissonance; we need more feeling, more resonance. I wish this for you.

Do you wish this for yourself? Are you interested in committing to disrupting dispositionalism in yourself and in this culture and seeking out who and what must be hidden to maintain a false sense of security? Are you willing to seek information and experiences that challenge you, not to make you stronger but to make you weaker, in right-proportion? Are you curious about your body, your intuition, all the magic the limbic system can bring to you? Can you feel in yourself the pull toward the complicated cracks and their gifts? Do you desire to be able to surrender to that pull? Can you sense the beginnings of the powerfully erotic in you? Do you want to be a witness as others sense their erotic power? Do you just have the slightest curiosity about the unraveling of worlds you can be part of? Will you hold all of us when you think of you and hold you when you think of all of us?

I invite you to mark this moment as a choice point. Being liberatory is remembering that oppression in this culture is easy, and it is never losing sight of that. It is recognizing oppression as a symptom of a culture that is analytical, logic-driven, time-obsessed, future-focused, honors the supremacy of innovation and glorifies the neocortex before it even targets a specific identity, place and/ or being. If your liberation begins with focusing on the targets, you've already missed it. Liberatory practice is not about what you do to or for others; it is about you and your seat as the practitioner.

Tayla writes of life as a love affair with the living body: "It requires a deep unwavering commitment to living life at the pace of the body, which is the pace of nature."[12] That is the invitation I am making to you. To make that deep unwavering commitment. It does not look any particular way; only you know if you are in or out of the commitment; it is not about discipline and perfectionism. Commitment means "always willing."

Will you be always willing?

Citations

1. Murphy, J. (2015). The therapeutic relationship in Hakomi therapy. In H. Weiss, L. Monda, & G. Johanson (Eds.), *Hakomi mindfulness-centered somatic psychotherapy: A comprehensive guide to theory and practice* (1st ed.). W.W. Norton & Company, Inc.

2. Owens, L. R. (2020). *Love and rage: The path of liberation through anger*. North Atlantic Books.

3. Haraway, D. J. (2016). *Staying with the trouble: Making Kin in the Chthulucene (experimental futures)* (Illustrated). Duke University Press Books.

4. Woodland, E., & Page, C. (2023). *Healing justice lineages: Dreaming at the crossroads of liberation, collective care, and safety*. North Atlantic Books.

5. Somé, M. P. (1997). *Ritual: Power, healing and community (compass)* (1st ed.). Penguin Books.

6. Johanson, G. (2015). Hakomi principles and a systems approach to psychotherapy. In H. Weiss, L. Monda, & G. Johanson (Eds.), *Hakomi mindfulness-centered somatic psychotherapy: A comprehensive guide to theory and practice* (1st ed.). W.W. Norton & Company, Inc.

7. Okawa, A. (2022, March 20). *#010: An invitation to a multicultural metatribe*. https://angellaokawa.substack.com/p/010-an-invitation-to-a-multicultural?s=w

8. Mesquita, B. (2022). *Between us: How cultures create emotions*. W. W. Norton & Company.

9. Lewis, T., Amini, F., & Lannon, R. (2001). *A general theory of love* (Reprint). Vintage.

10. Thanissara. (2015). *Time to stand up: An engaged Buddhist manifesto for our earth -- The Buddha's life and message through feminine eyes (sacred activism)* (1st ed.). North Atlantic Books.

11. Guggenbühl-Craig, A. (1996). *Power in the helping professions* (12th ed.). Spring Publications, Inc.

12. Shanaye, T. (2020). Nourishing the nervous system. Loam.

Index

For Product Safety Concerns and Information please contact our EU
representative GPSR@taylorandfrancis.com Taylor & Francis Verlag GmbH,
Kaufingerstraße 24, 80331 München, Germany

Printed and bound by CPI Group (UK) Ltd, Croydon, CR0 4YY
08/06/2025
01897005-0009